A Practical Guide for
**Aspiring
Ophthalmologists**

A Practical Guide for
Aspiring
Ophthalmologists

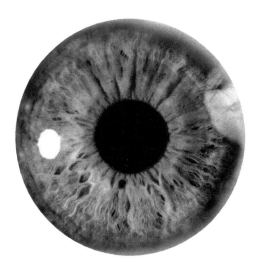

Sohaib R Rufai

NIHR Doctoral Fellow and Specialist Registrar in Ophthalmology
Great Ormond Street Hospital, UK

World Scientific

NEW JERSEY · LONDON · SINGAPORE · BEIJING · SHANGHAI · HONG KONG · TAIPEI · CHENNAI · TOKYO

Published by

World Scientific Publishing Co. Pte. Ltd.

5 Toh Tuck Link, Singapore 596224

USA office: 27 Warren Street, Suite 401-402, Hackensack, NJ 07601

UK office: 57 Shelton Street, Covent Garden, London WC2H 9HE

British Library Cataloguing-in-Publication Data
A catalogue record for this book is available from the British Library.

A PRACTICAL GUIDE FOR ASPIRING OPHTHALMOLOGISTS

ISBN 978-981-123-629-7 (hardcover)
ISBN 978-981-123-632-7 (paperback)
ISBN 978-981-123-630-3 (ebook for institutions)
ISBN 978-981-123-631-0 (ebook for individuals)

For any available supplementary material, please visit
https://www.worldscientific.com/worldscibooks/10.1142/12257#t=suppl

Disclaimer

This book is intended for candidates interested in applying for Ophthalmic Specialist Training (OST) in the UK. This book does not contain any shortcuts or secret insider information for the OST national recruitment process. Instead, this book contains guidance and strategies to aid preparation. This book is not affiliated to and does not represent the views of the Royal College of Ophthalmologists. The author accepts no responsibility for the use of the content of this book. Whilst every effort has been made to verify the content of this book, the author accepts no responsibility for any errors or omissions. Candidates are strongly advised to check the latest OST national recruitment guidance online provided by the Royal College of Ophthalmologists.

Contents

Dedication

This book was written in memory of my late grandfather, Noor-ud-Din Jeelani, Professor of Mathematics and first Vice-Chancellor of the University of Kashmir — a man who educated a nation.

This book was only possible thanks to the love and support of my wife, Tania, my parents, Shamim and Riyaz, my sisters, Sadaf and Shani, my supportive wider family and friends, plus my teachers who patiently guided me and encouraged me to work hard and dream big. I humbly dedicate this book to you all.

Foreword

Ophthalmology is a fascinating and fulfilling sub-speciality within medicine, not only because it deals with the diagnosis and treatment of disorders of such an important, discrete and highly evolved sensory organ, but also because it requires its practitioners to be polymaths.

The eye has been described in literature as the "window to the soul". In reality, it provides important clinical indicators of an individual's health because the clinician is uniquely able to examine in detail its internal structure and microvasculature without breaching its integrity.

Modern ophthalmologists require a broad range of skills encompassing medicine, surgery, optics, vision science and imaging techniques. Like other clinicians, ophthalmologists also benefit from holding strengths in evidence-based medicine and clinical research. Ophthalmology is certainly a field that provides huge opportunities in these areas. It is also an area of medicine that leads in the implementation of new technology. It has for decades been in the vanguard of the clinical utilisation of lasers, automated microsurgical techniques and cutting-edge imaging such as optical coherence tomography. More recently, ophthalmology has led the way in the use of artificial intelligence for improved diagnostic accuracy and the development of clinical algorithms. All this offers a rich vein of opportunities for both satisfying intellectual curiosity as well as, and more importantly, provision of the deep satisfaction that comes from helping patients.

It is a very busy speciality, one in which outpatient clinics and theatre lists are usually heavily booked. However, out of hours the work is not usually (outside the major conurbations) as heavy as in some of the more acute specialities. This can provide a measure of work-life balance for those who are not already irredeemable workaholics!

Ophthalmology has become increasingly popular and competitive in recent years. It enables its practitioners to provide both medical and surgical care to their patients and the opportunity to restore, stabilise or improve visual function, which is probably the most important sense that humans have.

Dr Sohaib Rufai is thus to be commended in producing this excellent book. He has provided a unique insight, drawn from his personal experience of ST training application, into what is required to successfully apply for ophthalmic training. The book outlines how to prepare for the application and the entry and selection criteria. He covers how to approach the MSRA computer-based test and the key points in producing an effective and comprehensive portfolio. He provides thorough guidance for preparation for the OST1 interview and helpful mock interview scenarios for practise.

To those of you reading this and thinking of applying to enter ophthalmic training, good luck with achieving your aim of a fantastic and fulfilling career. I unreservedly recommend this book, which contains sound advice and guidance to help you achieve that goal.

Professor I Christopher Lloyd, MB BS FRCS FRCOphth
Consultant Ophthalmic Surgeon and
Head of Ophthalmology,
Great Ormond Street Hospital for Children, London

About the Author

Dr Sohaib R. Rufai BMBS BMedSc MRes
Dr Rufai is an NIHR Doctoral Fellow and
Specialist Registrar (ST4) in Ophthalmology.
He works at Great Ormond Street Hospital
for Children, London.

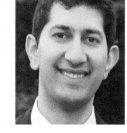

Dr Rufai has 30 peer-reviewed publications and 20 academic prizes from ARVO,
RCOphth, BIPOSA, BAAPS, MOS, the Ver-
non Trophy for Ophthalmological Research and others.

In 2014, Dr Rufai secured his first choice ophthalmology-themed NIHR Academic Foundation Post in Wessex. In 2016,
he was the number 1 ranked candidate in the UK's most competitive
NIHR Academic Clinical Fellowship ST1 post in Ophthalmology in
Leicester, during which he was awarded his MRes with distinction.
He led the world's first study using handheld optical coherence
tomography (OCT) to predict future vision in infantile nystagmus,
which was published in *Ophthalmology*, the highest impact clinical
journal in the field. In 2019, he was awarded a competitive NIHR
Doctoral Fellowship worth over £420,000 at Great Ormond Street
Hospital for Children. He secured all his posts on first attempt and
has helped numerous other successful OST1 applicants, many of
whom secured their top-ranked posts.

Endorsements

"This book reflects well the author's enthusiasm for ophthalmology and his effectiveness as a communicator. It is, above all, a practical and easy to access introduction into the life of a trainee ophthalmologist and should be a great help to anyone considering this career path."

Dr Frank Proudlock, Associate Professor of Ophthalmology, University of Leicester Ulverscroft Eye Unit

"Sohaib has been a tremendous help in the run-up to me being able to secure a highly competitive post in the North London Deanery, ranking 10th nationally. His advice and guidance allowed me to focus my preparation in high yield areas, which certainly paid off. I would recommend this book to anyone applying for ophthalmology training!"

Dr Abdullah Aamir, ST1, North London Deanery

"I just wanted to say a massive thanks to Sohaib for helping me get a post in Ophthalmology this year. His advice and teaching during my Ophthalmology rotation have truly been inspirational. From interview practice to building a competitive portfolio, Sohaib has really guided me and has opened many opportunities for me. I would highly recommend his book to all my fellow colleagues considering Ophthalmology as a career."

Dr Riddhi Thaker, ST1, West Midlands Deanery

"This is a great book, with very useful tips and I would recommend it to all applying for OST!"

Dr Swati Parida, ST1, East Midlands Deanery

1 Introduction

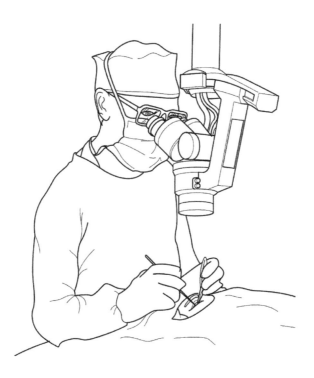

I should start by disclosing my significant bias towards ophthalmology as a career. I absolutely love ophthalmology. The art. The science. The lifestyle. The immense reward of improving a patient's vision. The attractive combination of medicine and surgery. Extremely high doctor and patient satisfaction. An arsenal of state-of-the-art technology at your disposal. Cutting-edge research. Favourable work-life balance. Probably the best job in the world, ever.

My interest in ophthalmology piqued when I was a third-year medical student at the University of Southampton. I remember attending an inspiring lecture titled "Tales of an Ophthalmologist", which was given by a highly personable and charismatic ophthalmologist. I asked this consultant if I could shadow him to learn more about the specialty, and he happily obliged. He would go on to become my supervisor for my intercalated BMedSc in ophthalmology. I led the undergraduate ophthalmology society at my university and organised ophthalmology seminars, skills sessions and conferences. I also arranged an ophthalmology-themed elective abroad, a further ophthalmology student-selected unit, and I got involved in several exciting projects. All this led to numerous presentations, publications and prizes while I completed medical school.

After graduating, I completed an ophthalmology-themed NIHR Academic Foundation Post in Southampton and NIHR Academic Clinical Fellowship (ST1–3) in ophthalmology in Leicester. I am currently an NIHR Doctoral Fellow and Specialist Registrar (ST4) at Great Ormond Street Hospital, London. I was extremely fortunate to secure these posts on my first attempt, which is a testament to the foresight and guidance of my mentors.

Looking back, I feel that the key to getting into ophthalmic specialist training (OST) was being enthusiastic and persistent and seeking guidance from those in a position to help me. I find most ophthalmologists tend to be friendly and helpful people, so when they come across an enthusiastic student/junior doctor showing a genuine interest in their specialty, they usually try to help wherever they can. By simply getting involved and becoming known in the department, opportunities kept presenting themselves, and I managed to get my foot in the door.

I am truly privileged to have discovered ophthalmology as a career option relatively early on. Since securing my own OST1 post, I am delighted to have helped numerous candidates successfully secure their OST1 posts, of whom many were awarded their first-choice posts. While delivering my coaching and preparatory sessions, my students and peers strongly encouraged me to write this book to share the knowledge and experience that I have gained first-hand from each step of this journey. Even if you have decided to pursue ophthalmology later on in your career, you can still succeed in securing a training post, provided you take the right steps and prepare well.

In this book, I want to help you achieve your dream career in ophthalmology. I also hope to share my passion with you for this wonderful specialty.

2 A Week in the Life of an Ophthalmology Trainee

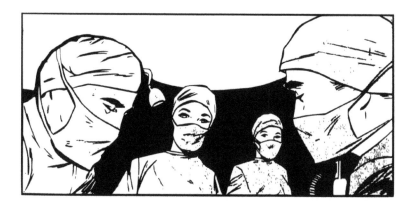

Ophthalmology is truly a craft specialty. As such, close supervision and guidance in the early stages are essential for mastering your craft. You may be reassured to learn that you will typically start off watching things from the passenger seat in your first moments as a fledgling ST1. Next, you may be given a reduced clinic to allow your consultant or senior colleague to review your patients a second time. As you build experience, your consultant or senior colleague may simply listen to you present your patient and agree upon a management plan. Eventually, you will be able to see most of your patients yourself with occasional senior input where needed.

A typical day is divided into two sessions: morning (AM) and afternoon (PM). These sessions typically could include clinic, theatre, eye casualty, laser, injections, minor ops, regional teaching and self-directed RSTA (Research, Study, Teaching and Audit). Clinics could be general or specialist, depending on your training stage and location.

On-calls tend to work a bit differently in ophthalmology from what you may be used to in other jobs. Although some large eye units have night shift rotas, it is far more common to do non-resident on-call (NROC) shifts after hours. This means you can leave the hospital and take urgent calls from home, usually until the following morning. There is typically a two- or three-tier on call system depending on location, meaning that if you are the first on call, there will be someone more senior also on call for you to seek help from (and possibly someone more senior for that person to seek help from if operating a three-tier system). It is not unusual to start off discussing most of your calls with your senior colleague before deciding your plan. Your senior colleague may also attend and review the patient with you, depending on the situation. Junior trainees will typically attend in person to see a greater proportion of referrals, while more senior trainees typically may have the experience to safely manage more patients with advice over the phone and arrange reviews where necessary. Weekends on call will usually involve seeing urgent patients during the day, followed by NROCs after hours and overnight.

To give you a flavour, here is a fairly typical weekly rota for an ophthalmology trainee (with the NROC falling on alternate weeks after 17:30 until 08:30 the following morning):

A Typical OST Weekly Rota

Mon AM	Clinic
Mon PM	Laser
Tue AM	Clinic
Tue PM	Eye Casualty (and NROC on alternate weeks)
Wed AM	RSTA
Wed PM	Theatre
Thur AM	Clinic
Thur PM	RSTA
Fri AM	Theatre
Fri PM	Regional teaching
Weekends	1 in 6

And there you have it — an exciting week in the life of an ophthalmology trainee. The clinical workload can get very busy, but on balance I feel the rewards of the job far outweigh the drawbacks.

If you have decided that this career appeals to you, the challenging part is getting through the highly competitive national selection process and landing a training post. In the rest of this book, I aim to boost your chances of success at each step of your journey.

3 Am I Suited to Ophthalmology?

Chapter

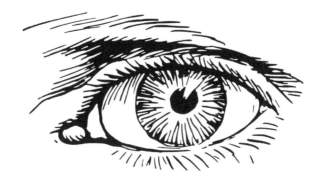

To truly figure out whether ophthalmology is a suitable career for you, there is no substitute for seeing what the job entails first-hand. Find a friendly ophthalmologist who can help arrange shadowing or taster experience in the department and take it from there. Attending ophthalmology conferences or seminars can also help you decide. As far as the OST1 application is concerned, there are essential and desirable criteria outlined within the Person Specification. Another tool currently used to select suitable candidates is the Multi-Specialty Recruitment Assessment (MSRA). This chapter will provide a brief overview of both.

Person Specification

The OST1 Person Specification is available online via the Severn Postgraduate Medical Education Resources (Severn PGME,

9

2020a). This guide provides the essential criteria, desirable criteria and details for when each criterion is evaluated, e.g. application form, interview/selection centre, references, etc. You should read through these criteria carefully. Here is a very brief overview of what sort of criteria are assessed, as per the 2021 Person Specification (Severn PGME, 2020a):

- Entry criteria
  - Qualifications
  - Eligibility
  - Fitness to practise
  - Language skills
  - Health
  - Career progression
  - Application completion
- Selection criteria
  - Qualifications
  - Clinical skills — clinical knowledge and expertise
  - Academic skills
  - Personal skills
  - Probity — professional integrity
  - Commitment to specialty — learning and personal development

Again, ensure that you read through the official Person Specification carefully, which contains subsections and full details of essential and desirable criteria. You should aim to fulfil the latter to boost your chances of a successful application.

Multi-Specialty Recruitment Assessment (MSRA)

The Multi-Specialty Recruitment Assessment (MSRA) is a computer-based test delivered in partnership with the Work Psychology

Group and Pearson VUE (Severn PGME, 2020a). It is designed to assess essential competencies based around clinical scenarios. There are two sections in the MSRA: Professional Dilemmas and Clinical Problem Solving. You will need to refer to the official guidance and seek suitable preparation resources for the MSRA, as this falls outside the scope of this book.

As per the 2020 OST1 guidance, all eligible applicants for OST1 will be invited to sit for the MSRA. A minimum score in the MSRA is required to be invited for an interview. Furthermore, the MSRA contributes a maximum of 40 points, which represent 20% of the 200 points (portfolio: 100 points; interview stations: 160 points; MSRA: 40 points) available in total. This means that the higher your MSRA score is, the higher the chances of you securing an OST1 post. Therefore, it is worth investing ample time and effort in preparing for the MSRA. Please do check the most up to date OST1 guidance online, as the scoring can change from year to year. *Please note — the updated 2021 OST1 guidance has changed as follows: MSRA — 20 points; Evidence Folder — 50 points; Online Assessment (Interview) — 30 points.*

The Professional Dilemmas section is in many ways similar to the Situational Judgment Test (SJT) taken by medical students prior to commencing the Foundation Programme. This section covers three core areas: professional integrity, coping with pressure, and empathy and sensitivity. This section assesses professional behaviour and situational judgment, rather than specific clinical knowledge. The question types include ranking (in order of "appropriateness") and multiple-choice questions.

The Clinical Problem Solving section assesses your application of medical knowledge and clinical decision-making. The questions could relate to any of the body systems, so a broad approach to revision is key. This section assesses areas including investigation, diagnosis, prescribing, clinical management, medical emergencies and more. The question types include extended matching questions and single best answer questions.

Again, it is worth investing ample time into your MSRA preparation. Treat this exam with the same attention and respect as your medical school exams. Look through the official guidance and plan a structured revision timetable. You will be surprised how quickly you can turn your weaknesses into strengths once you have understood the material well. Question banks are available online to aid your preparation — speak to colleagues and check reviews before subscribing. Look for patterns in the questions you answer incorrectly and try to diagnose and treat the underlying problem, which can often fall into one of these four categories: (i) depth of understanding, (ii) breadth of understanding, (iii) the need to consolidate knowledge, and (iv) suboptimal exam technique (including failure to read the question properly). Don't worry that the general medical knowledge you are learning for the MSRA is "going to waste" just because you are pursuing a career in ophthalmology. Ophthalmologists are doctors too and are often the first to pick up systemic diseases manifesting in the eye. Just think, a seemingly trivial piece of medical knowledge you learned for this exam may change or save a patient's life in the future.

4 The Evidence Folder

Chapter

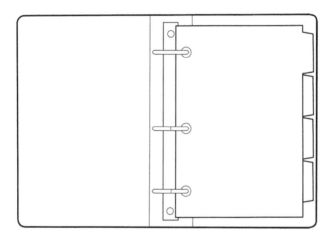

Please note: *This information is in line with the 2021 OST1 national recruitment guidance. Certain aspects may change over time. Please ensure that you check the latest requirements via the Royal College of Ophthalmologists website (RCOphth, 2020a).*

Overview

The evidence folder, also known as the "portfolio of evidence", is a great source of points within the application process. The earlier you start building a strong evidence folder, the higher your chances of maximising these precious points. Try to see this as an opportunity for learning and growth, and don't forget to have fun along the way!

Prior to the new 2021 OST application guidelines, candidates were required to produce and hand over a physical folder containing all their evidence to the interview panel. However, for the 2021 application cycle, due to COVID-19 precautions, applicants must upload their documentation onto an online evidence portal. Full information for the 2021 application cycle, including a link to the evidence portal, will be provided to candidates prior to the portal opening on 18 January 2021. The deadline to upload this documentation is 29 January 2021.

I recommend starting a list of "Portfolio Goals" early, in which you can list the points you already have, followed by your goals for scoring additional points with target timelines. We will look at strategies for boosting your score later in this chapter.

This is the evidence folder's list of contents with a scoring guide per section, as per the 2021 OST1 national recruitment guidance (Severn PGME, 2020a). Again, please ensure that you check the latest guidance as some aspects may change over time. It is extremely important to provide the evidence requested per section, as no points will be awarded for incorrect or missing evidence.

OST1 Portfolio Contents

Section	Criteria	Points
Previous Posts		
List of Previous Posts	Previous posts in reverse chronological order	N/A
Education		
Qualifications	Cumulative scoring with a maximum of 4 points. Certificates or letters of evidence required.	
	PhD/DPhil	3 points
	MD thesis	2 points
	Undergraduate or masters level qualification, e.g., intercalated BSc, BA, MSc	1 point
Prizes/Awards	Cumulative scoring with a maximum of 5 points.	
	1st in undergraduate degree	1 point
	Best paper or presentation at international meeting	2 points
	Crombie medal for standing 1st in FRCOphth Part 1	2 points
	National undergraduate prize (in any specialty), e.g., The Duke Elder Prize: 2 points for the top 10% of entrants; 1 point for the top 60% of entrants.	1–2 points
	Best paper or poster at a national meeting	1 point

(Continued)

(Continued)

	Successful research grant application	1 point
Training and Experience		
Ophthalmology Specialty Links and Commitment To Date as a Career	Cumulative scoring with a maximum of 12 points.	
	FRCOphth Part 1	3 points
	Refraction Certificate	2 points
	Case report / Non peer-reviewed publication as first author, e.g., published in undergraduate journals	1 point (4 points max.)
	Attendance at national or international ophthalmology meeting or course	1 point (2 points max.)
	Attendance at regional ophthalmology meeting	0.5 point (1 point max.)
	Ophthalmic elective/project	1 point (max.)
	RCOphth Introduction to Ophthalmic Surgery course	1 point
	EyeSi assessments (minimum 4 hours)	1 point (max.)
	Presentations at undergraduate meetings	1 point

(Continued)

	Attendance in eye clinic and theatre sessions (10 sessions minimum with dates — signed evidence required)	1 point (max.)
Multi-Source Feedback (MSF)	Must be within 18 months prior to an interview date. Standard Team Assessment Behaviour Form (TAB) from Foundation Programme Horus E-Portfolio can be included without a signature or departmental stamp. For other candidates, please seek guidance via the OST1 National Recruitment website.	5 points max.
Audit, Research and Training		
Publications	List of publications — original articles or studies with a copy of the first page included. No marks are awarded without any copy of the first page or evidence of the accepted paper. Completed publications proforma must be included (see below*)	5 points max.

(Continued)

(Continued)

Quality Improvement/ Audit Projects	Include your best quality improvement (QI) or audit project. Must be within three years prior to an interview date. The audit must have standards, outcomes and recommendations. Must be signed by a supervising consultant. A cover letter or certificate is required for proof of presentation.	5 points max.
Presentations	Cumulative scoring with a maximum of 6 points. List your presentations with copies of abstracts or posters, stating whether they are oral or poster presentations. Must include a copy of an abstract book or signed letter from a supervisor as evidence. The same study presented at different meetings will only be scored once at the highest-ranking meeting.	
	International meeting	3 points
	National meeting	2 points
	Regional meeting	1 point
Education and Teaching	Cumulative scoring with a maximum of 5 points.	

(Continued)

	Higher teaching qualification, e.g., Masters, diploma or certificate in medical education; writing a book; writing a textbook chapter; formal role in examining undergraduates; teaching the teacher course; or designing an educational course or e-learning tool.	5 points max.
Overall Portfolio Layout and Quality		
Global Quality and Presentation	Assessment of layout, organisation and quality of presentation.	3 points max.

*The publication proforma can be downloaded from the Evidence Folder webpage on the Severn Deanery website. (Severn PGME, 2020a) A link for Cite-Factor is also provided on the same webpage, which is used to determine the impact factor of the journal. For each included publication, the impact factor is multiplied by the authorship score, which is assigned as follows:

- 1st author: 4 points
- 2nd author: 3 points
- 3rd author: 2 points
- 4th author or beyond: 1 point

For example, below is a candidate who has one original research study published in the journal *Eye*.

OST1 Publication Proforma — Example

Name of Journal	Impact Factor	Authorship Score	Impact Factor x Authorship Score
Example: *Eye*	2.478	4 (1st author)	9.912
Total Score			9.912

Before we move on, I want to reassure you of a few things:

1. Don't feel overwhelmed. Plan goals for each section. If you managed to get through medical school, you already possess the initiative and organisational skills to put together a good portfolio.
2. Building your portfolio is a marathon, not a sprint. It will not happen overnight. Give yourself plenty of time.
3. Remember that some of these criteria will help candidates who took longer routes to get here, such as previous academics with PhDs or teaching qualifications. Only a minority of foundation doctors who studied medicine as a first degree will have these additional higher degrees.
4. You will have several other opportunities to score points, namely the interview and the MSRA.

Next, we will look at strategies for you to maximise your score, including easy wins, by simply planning ahead and taking the right steps.

Maximising Your Portfolio Score

There are plenty of opportunities to score a lot of the points on the portfolio with relative ease. The key is forward planning and ensuring that you collect all the low hanging fruit. Some points may be more difficult to achieve during the COVID-19 pandemic. However you secure the points, each point brings you a step closer to your dream career in ophthalmology. I will go through each section and suggest strategies you can use to boost your score.

Qualifications

It is difficult to quickly pick up points in this section. If you are still a medical student and have the option to do an intercalated degree, this would give you an extra point and nurture you with opportunities to score multiple points across the rest of the portfolio. More importantly, an intercalated degree could ignite your passion for that subject. If you are reapplying for ophthalmology ST1 and do not have an intercalated degree, some candidates opt for studying a relevant master's degree while working on whichever areas of their portfolio were weaker in their previous application. This often leads to a successful reapplication.

Don't worry if you don't have a PhD/DPhil. These points reward the experience of previous academics with careers prior to medicine (hence, very rare for those coming straight out of undergraduate medicine and the Foundation Programme!) There are some opportunities for medical students to combine their medical degree and PhD before even starting the Foundation Programme. However, I would only advocate the pursuit of a PhD at such an early stage if you are truly passionate about researching a particular area and not just to score a few points on this application. Completing a PhD is a long, hard road. Plus, there are many advantages to studying for a PhD later on in your career, especially as a funded doctoral fellow where you can have more autonomy over your project, more training opportunities and a higher salary compared to those on standard PhD studentships.

Prizes and awards

This is also not the easiest section for quickly picking up points. However, if you are a medical student, it is worth sitting the Duke Elder exam as you are given 1 point for scoring within the top 60% of candidates, which is achievable with good preparation. If you work really hard you may even score well enough to be within the top 10% and achieve 2 points here.

As for the presentation prizes, you will first need to identify suitable target conferences for the work you have produced and wish to present. Your supervisor and senior colleagues can help advise you. Look at previous winning examples, which are often posted online on the conference website. Attend conferences and observe which presentations win a prize — reflect on why you think that presentation/work was the best and how you can emulate these characteristics in your presentation/work where applicable. Another tip is to diversify your presentations, for example, poster and oral, or different conference specialties or even different categories within the same conference. Seek feedback each time from supervisors and seniors on how to improve.

Another important tip for winning prizes — you must aim to win. It is extremely rare for anybody to accidentally win anything. However, as per the Law of Attraction, if you adopt a positive mind-set, work hard and visualise yourself winning a competition, you are far more likely to win the competition. Of course, there is a huge amount of luck involved and it can be very unpredictable with these sorts of prizes. If at first you don't succeed, try, try again. With hard work and perseverance, it is entirely possible to win a prize during the junior years of your career.

If you can get a 1st in your undergraduate degree, you get another point. (Don't beat yourself up if you don't win the Crombie Medal for standing 1st in the FRCOphth Part 1!)

Ophthalmology specialty links and commitment

Normally, this section is full of low-hanging fruit. However, some of these points may be more difficult to access during the COVID-19 pandemic. Alas, these are the guidelines set by the powers that be. Undertaking a taster week in ophthalmology gets you 1 point. Attending ten sessions in the eye department gets you 1 point. Attending the RCOphth Introduction to Ophthalmic Surgery course gets you 1 point. A presentation at an undergraduate meeting gets you 1 point. Attending two national meetings and two regional meetings gets you 3 points. Please note: many of these meetings have been converted to virtual delivery due to COVID-19, so these may be easier to achieve in some cases.

If you arrange to use an EyeSi (an ophthalmic surgical simulator), you can score 1 point just for using it for four hours. They are extremely useful for developing microsurgical skills and are good fun too. The Royal College of Ophthalmologists has compiled a list of EyeSi simulators around the UK and Ireland with contact details (RCOphth, 2020b).

If possible, you can try to arrange an ophthalmology elective or project for another point. Whatever your stage, if you show enthusiasm and commitment to a friendly ophthalmologist near you, they may allow you to write case reports, letters to the editor or an article in a non peer-reviewed journal. More importantly, establishing a good relationship with an ophthalmologist can help you score points across a wide range of the portfolio, understand the specialty better and generally enrich your life for the better.

At this point, I should highlight that these electives, courses and meetings usually cost money and involve associated travel unless delivered virtually. However, consider this an investment today into your dream career as an ophthalmologist tomorrow. There are usually discounted rates for trainees at meetings, and some meetings are even free for trainees. You can also use study budget, if available, or apply for various travel bursaries to help. When I was a medical student, I got into two national conferences for free by offering to help pass the microphone around during the Q&A sessions. This may have been an uncommon arrangement, but if you don't ask, you don't get!

Finally, the FRCOphth Part 1 is a challenging exam that takes several months of committed preparation. It would certainly not fall within the "low-hanging fruit" category. It is worth 3 points if you pass, but there are numerous other points in this section that are a safer bet. However, if you feel you can invest adequate time preparing for this exam without losing the other points, then go for it. I must say, I am surprised to see the Refraction Certificate in this section, but if you somehow become proficient in refraction (or are a qualified optometrist) and pass the Refraction Exam, then you earn another 2 points.

Multi-Source Feedback (MSF)

The best way to score many points here is to strive to be a good colleague. It is a joy to work with someone who is well mannered and considerate; these qualities seldom go unnoticed. Try to write down and memorise everyone's names whenever you start a new job and ask them how they are doing; they will notice and appreciate this.

Try to help out with rota swaps and covering sickness where possible. Some people become "extra nice" around the time of their MSF, but it is better to commit to good habits and behaviour all year round to build positive working relationships with the wider team. This ultimately makes your life easier too!

Publications

It used to be exceptionally rare for a medical student or junior doctor to publish papers. Alas, for better or worse, there is more emphasis placed on publishing papers these days. It is not impossible to get a post without scoring any points in the publications section, but the points would have to be compensated for elsewhere.

Ideally, publications should stem from being actively involved within a department, taking a genuine interest in the subject and conducting a project that advances science and contributes genuine value. However, another type of publication stems from publishing for the sake of publication, or people trying to get their names on papers with minimal input, purely to get points on application forms. This is not unique to ophthalmology but more or less across the board. Many people fall into the latter category in a bid to secure a training post, where there is so much emphasis on publications. However, "bad science" must be avoided at all costs!

I would highly encourage the route of engaging closely with a research group or department and showing a keen interest in their field. Candidates may have formal time and supervisors allocated for research, such as those doing an intercalated degree or Academic Foundation Post. However, in my experience, all one needs to do is spend time in the department to get your face known, approach a potential supervisor, express a genuine interest in their field, and direct or indirect opportunities will eventually come your way. First-author publication opportunities come with effective networking, enthusiasm and hard work.

The best person to help you conduct your project is your supervisor. They should be able to guide you with relevant literature to read, research question formulation, data collection, data analysis and then making sense of it all. When it comes to writing a paper, I find the following approach helpful:

1. Draft a *Title* to convey the main area(s) that your study addresses.
2. Write your *Results* section first. Design tables and figures where applicable to help the data tell a story and convey a clear message.
3. Write your *Methods* section such that the order logically leads on to your *Results* section.
4. Write the *Introduction* concisely and logically to set the scene for the *Methods* section, including the research questions/objectives.
5. Write the *Discussion* next, which should cover the key results, put the results into context of existing literature, and address the strengths and limitations. This should be followed by the conclusion.
6. Write the *Abstract* next, summarising the background, methods, results and conclusion.
7. Finalise your *Title*, ensuring it addresses the main area(s) of the paper.

This is just my personal approach and may not suit everyone. I realised that once the *Results* section is done, everything else tends to fall into place and the paper becomes more enjoyable to write. I also found that I spent less time going back and re-writing previous sections to restore the flow of the paper. However, it is completely up to the individual on how they wish to approach writing a paper, but the most important thing is to produce "good science". Ensure that you follow the journal's guidelines and use appropriate checklists depending on the study type. Critical appraisal is covered in The In-Person Interview chapter.

Just a final tip on publications: if you are really struggling to get started on a research study with barriers including ethical approval and so forth, a good alternative would be to conduct a systematic review. This requires no ethical approval and you can hit the ground running. *The Cochrane Handbook for Systematic Reviews of Interventions* is freely available online (Cochrane, 2020). All you need is a good topic to review and a second person to screen the literature with you — your supervisor can help you identify both. A well-conducted systematic review on an important topic can produce an incredibly valuable paper and is likely to get published. Just make sure that the topic is not so broad that you end up with mountains of literature to screen with no end in sight. The key is to formulate a specific and important clinical question.

Quality improvement/audit

You can only include one quality improvement (QI) or audit project in this section, and it should be conducted within three years of the interview date. There is a maximum of 5 points, and the scoring is at the discretion of the judging panel. Please see the Improving Patient Care section within The In-Person Interview chapter for detailed information on approaching QI and audit.

Presentations

This is a relatively straightforward section to collect points. Typically, it is much easier to get an abstract accepted at a conference than to publish a paper. Many conferences have switched to virtual delivery since the COVID-19 pandemic, thus making it easier for participants to attend regional, national or even international conferences. Note that the same presentation at different meetings will only be counted once at the highest-ranking meeting.

A good tactic would be to ensure all your smaller projects, such as smaller-scale audits, QI projects or even case reports, get presented at least at regional meetings (1 point). Ask a friendly consultant or senior colleague about which regional meetings may be suitable. As for national (2 points) versus international (3 points) conferences, I would recommend aiming for the latter wherever possible for more substantial projects to maximise your score. For example, the RCOphth Congress, the Association for Research in Vision and Ophthalmology (ARVO) and the American Academy of Ophthalmology annual meetings count as international meetings. Equivalent non-ophthalmology meetings also count. In terms of in-person meetings, factor in the travel cost involved. However, if you have the necessary travel funds, there are plenty of excellent meetings in Europe and beyond that often offer discounts for students and trainees.

If you have never presented work before, it is helpful to attend a meeting and observe others presenting oral presentations or posters. You can even approach the presenters when the time is right and ask them questions, including how they conducted their project and put together their slides or poster, tips for getting started, etc. Read example abstracts in conference abstract books available online to familiarise yourself with the content and format required. Conferences usually provide clear guidelines for the required abstract structure as well as oral presentations and posters — ensure that you read these very carefully. There is usually someone who turns up with the wrong sized poster — don't be that person...

For oral presentations, consider visiting the venue in advance to familiarise yourself with the stage and setup. For instance, where will you be sitting? What is the route to the stage? Are there stairs? Is there a radio microphone, handheld microphone, or is the microphone attached to a podium? Will a clicker or laser pointer be provided? The principle of visiting early also applies to virtual presentations — ensure that you have access to the correct platform and that your video and audio are all in working order. Have a practice run using the virtual platform to get comfortable before the real thing.

In terms of slide design, there are usually guidelines provided by the meeting organiser. The aim is to translate your scientific abstract (typically including the background, methods, results and conclusions) into slide format in an engaging and informative presentation. To avoid overrunning, aim for approximately two slides per minute. Avoid too much text on your slides — try to stick to a maximum of 25–30 words. Opt for clear, sans serif fonts (such as Calibri) as these are easier to read when enlarged/resized, as opposed to serif fonts (such as Times New Roman), which look better in print. Include images where possible — make sure they are labelled for reuse if sourced online or that you have full permission to use them. Reformat or redesign your figures so that they can be easily read and interpreted in slide format.

In terms of presenting your slides — practise, practise, practise. Deliver your presentation to your supervisor, colleagues, friends and family. Take their feedback on board. Keep calm. Staying calm is a superpower. Figure out a good routine (for example, using mindfulness, breathing exercises, pep talk or whatever technique works for you) that will help you stay cool, calm and collected. Consider scripting your opening lines. Practise in front of a mirror if that is helpful. Plan your outfit several days in advance. Wear clothes that make you feel confident. Walk tall to the stage and deliver your polished opening line with confidence and open body language. Keep your head up and engage with your audience. Use eye contact to keep them engaged. If it is a smaller audience, you can make eye contact at an individual level and vary this to engage every audience member at various times. If it is a very large audience, you can direct your talk to different segments of the audience at different times to keep everyone engaged. Own the stage. If you have a handheld or radio microphone, consider walking around the stage to speak to different segments of the audience — motivational speakers and comedians often use this technique to engage the audience. If the microphone is attached to a podium, you can still vary the direction you face through your talk to address different segments of the audience. If your talk is conducted virtually, then be sure to make eye contact with the camera. Remember, you are the presenter and your slides come secondary to you. The focus of the presentation should be you, while the slides act as a backdrop.

When it comes to answering questions — again, keep calm. A good way to anticipate likely questions is by practising with colleagues and peers and noting the pattern of questions that arises — this can steer your responses towards the areas you are familiar with, especially if the question seems less relevant. If you don't know the answer, graciously admit that the questioner has raised an interesting point that you have not covered in your project, which you can take back to your supervisor and team to explore further.

When it comes to posters, the format is slightly different. The aim is to translate your scientific abstract into an engaging and informative poster format. A good poster should not only work well as your backdrop during your allocated poster session when you present to audience members and judges but also function as a stand-alone source of information for conference attendees roaming around during coffee breaks. Many conferences opt for ePosters, whether in person or virtual. A good poster should have clear figures that are easy to interpret. Avoid being too wordy or using small font sizes. Again, opt for sans serif fonts, as these are easier to read when resized. Also, avoid colour templates or obscure fonts that make your poster difficult to read. Show your draft poster to your supervisor and peers to seek feedback and improve wherever possible. Poster sessions can stimulate great discussion and debate, as you may only be interacting with a small number of people or only one person at a time. This can improve your project and paper writing immensely, as you can effectively receive peer review of your work from a variety of audience members. Relish the opportunity to present your work in either oral or poster format and enjoy the ride.

Education and teaching

Perhaps the easiest win in this section is completing a teach the teacher course. You can check online for suitable courses. The rest of the points in this section will require a bit more initiative.

If you are a doctor interested in a formal role in examining undergraduate students, such as objective structured clinical examinations (OSCEs), contact your local medical school to see what opportunities there are. As a medical student, this may be difficult unless you are permitted to examine mock exams in younger years, for example. Ideally, you can be formally appointed an examiner for the medical school after you graduate.

A good approach to organising an educational course would be to team up with a few colleagues and decide on a topic that you would feel comfortable delivering teaching for and where there is a need. For example, you could organise a regional teaching course for medical students preparing for their finals or OSCEs. You could approach friendly consultants to deliver some of the content/ sessions with you. They can also sign a letter of evidence for your portfolio. If you want the course to be professional, you could even produce a course handbook/booklet with clear learning objectives per session, assessing the student's confidence and abilities before and after the course. It may even be possible to publish your find-ings to share your methods if your course is novel and demon-strates a significant impact on learning. Be sure to collect feedback to reflect on how to improve your teaching.

With regards to e-learning tools, you can be creative with these. They could even complement the educational course(s) you deliver to help your students consolidate their learning. One example could be a video tutorial for medical students. First, you would need to decide on the topic, such as a specific OSCE exam-ination or overview of a subject for exam revision. Ideally, you should show the video to a consultant or appropriate assessor first to ensure the content is suitable. Then, you can upload this to an online platform, such as YouTube. Ask a medical school admin-istrator for advice or assistance with disseminating your content to the relevant students. You could even screenshot the webpage showing your video and the associated number of "views" and/or feedback in the comments section. You can also ask your supervi-sor to date and sign the page to confirm that it is your work. If you are technologically savvy, you could produce interactive e-learning resources such as pharmacology mind maps, interactive anatomy models and acute medicine simulation storyboards — the sky is the limit. If you have great ideas but are unsure on how to produce the resource, find someone in the medical school or beyond who could help you to produce this.

The remaining criteria are relatively difficult to achieve quickly, such as writing a book or a chapter in a textbook. A higher teaching qualification will also take considerable time. However, if you have a real passion for medical education, a diploma or masters in medical education may be an attractive option for you. For candidates taking a year out to re-apply for OST1, this could also represent a valuable experience in the interim.

Global quality and presentation

Finally, there are 3 marks available for the layout, organisation and quality of presentation of your portfolio of evidence. This score is down to the discretion of the judging panel. For the 2021 application cycle, it is unclear how these marks will be allocated for the virtual evidence uploaded to the online portal. Every single document in your evidence folder should be included with the aim of scoring points, as per the official guidance. Only include documentation that has been requested and do not include any unnecessary information as this could risk losing marks. If possible, ask a consultant or senior colleague familiar with the OST1 portfolio if they could look at yours for feedback.

In case the physical portfolio is brought back, make sure your portfolio is not overly bulky or cluttered as this could lose marks. Put yourself in the shoes of the judges who will spend hours looking through a large series of portfolios. The easier you make it for them to go through and mark your portfolio, the more likely you are to score these points. Try to make it a pleasure to go through your portfolio. Structure your portfolio as per the official guidance and you should ideally use dividers for the relevant sections. Check that you can turn all the pages smoothly; otherwise, it is probably overfilled. Invest in good quality, A4-punched pocket sleeves and ensure that you get a ring binder with four rings as this allows for smoother page turning. Don't lose too much sleep over what ring binder to purchase — as long as it looks tidy and professional, you should be fine.

Debrief

This may seem like a lot to get through, but provided you give yourself enough time and approach this systematically, you can significantly boost your score. Try to break it down into individual sections and list the things you have already scored points for. Then, write down your "Portfolio Goals" with realistic timelines. It is helpful to do this in a Word document so that you can edit as you go along. The key is to plan ahead, including organising your leave for relevant courses and meetings. Start early and don't forget to enjoy the journey. This is your opportunity to learn, showcase your achievements and shine.

5 The Online Interview (2021)

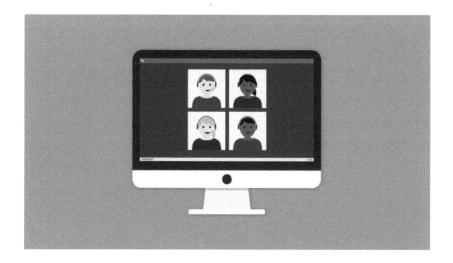

Please note: *Due to the COVID-19 pandemic, the 2021 OST interviews will be delivered virtually via Microsoft Teams. At the time of writing, it is unclear whether this will be a long-term format or whether the interviews will revert to the traditional "in-person" format in the future. Hence, this book contains chapters for both formats, with a degree of overlap between the two. Please ensure that you check the latest requirements via the Royal College of Ophthalmologists website (RCOphth, 2020a).*

General Information

OST1 recruitment has been centralised since 2012 and is co-ordinated by the Severn Deanery. Due to the COVID-19 pandemic, the 2021 OST interviews will be delivered online via Microsoft Teams. At the time of writing, the 2021 interview date is advertised as 12 March 2021 (RCOphth, 2020a).

The online interview will take the format of a patient consultation and will involve conversing with an actor. The initial identity checks, interview and debrief will take approximately 30 minutes in total. *Please note — the updated 2021 OST guidance advises that candidates have 3 minutes for preparation and 7 minutes for the patient consultation (interview) with the actor.*

This is an unprecedented situation. The guidance available from Severn PGME (2020a) is relatively brief; it simply describes the interview format as a "patient consultation". Therefore, a safe and sensible strategy would be to thoroughly prepare communication skills and clinical knowledge to boost your chances of success and avoid getting caught out. Being overprepared is better than being underprepared. Ensure your personal computer has good audiovisual functionality and consider using a headset if this significantly improves your audio quality.

This chapter will offer strategies for preparing your communication skills and clinical knowledge to a high standard.

Communication Skills

There is increasing importance placed on effective communication skills within undergraduate and postgraduate medical training. OST interviews are no exception — in fact, this is well justified as good communication is particularly important in a field as specialised as ophthalmology.

The patient consultation might involve delivering medical information, addressing knowledge gaps, providing reassurance, speaking to an angry or upset patient/relative, breaking bad news, or a combination thereof. Please note that this list is not exhaustive — in theory, any scenario testing your communication skills could come up. It is therefore important to train well and hone your communication skills across a wide variety of practice scenarios.

You may find techniques covered in the Calgary–Cambridge framework (Kurtz *et al.*, 2003) helpful for approaching the patient consultation. Please note that this framework normally applies to the full medical consultation (such as for general practice), whereas your OST interview scenario may only deal with specific aspects. Your scenario might focus more on information gathering and explanation rather than decision-making, but there could be an element of the latter as well. These are the key elements within the enhanced Calgary–Cambridge framework (Kurtz *et al.*, 2003):

- Initiating the session
  - Preparation
  - Establishing rapport
  - Identifying reasons for the consultation
- Gathering information
  - Explore the patient's problem to discover:
    - Biomedical perspective
    - Patient's perspective
    - Background information (context)
- Physical examination (not applicable here)
- Explanation and planning
  - Provide the correct amount and type of information
  - Aid accurate recall and understanding
  - Achieve a shared understanding
  - Planning — shared decision-making
- Closing the session
  - Ensuring appropriate point of closure
  - Forward planning

The Calgary–Cambridge framework (Kurtz *et al.*, 2003) also includes process skills for exploration of the patient's problems:

- Patient's narrative
- Questioning style: open to closed
- Attentive listening
- Facilitative response
- Picking up cues
- Clarification
- Time-framing
- Internal summary
- Appropriate language
- Additional skills for understanding the patient's perspective

Finally, the enhanced Calgary–Cambridge framework (Kurtz *et al.*, 2003) also includes a suggested structure for exploring the biomedical perspective, patient's perspective and background information:

- Biomedical perspective (disease)
  - Sequence of events
  - Symptoms analysis
  - Relevant systems review
- Patient's perspective (illness)
  - ICE: ideas, concerns and expectations
  - Effects on life
  - Feelings
- Background information (context)
  - Past medical history
  - Drug history and allergies
  - Family history
  - Personal and social history
  - Review of systems

The RAV model is another model you may find helpful for demonstrating empathy (Marsden, 2014):

- **Recognise** that a patient has an emotional response to a situation, detecting their verbal and nonverbal cues;
- **Acknowledge** this emotional response;
- **Validate** their emotional response with empathy.

An example could be a patient who seems visibly distressed when you talk about intravitreal injections. You **recognise** that their body language has changed from previously being relaxed to now wincing and recoiling. You can **acknowledge** their emotional response by pausing and using a phrase such as: "I can see you seem distressed when I mention injections — is that right?" The patient may then reply in the affirmative. Then, you can **validate** their response with a phrase such as: "I understand that this may sound frightening to you at first — your reaction is quite natural and not uncommon." You can follow this up by exploring the patient's concerns and fears, reassuring them and being supportive. Partnership statements can also be helpful, such as "we will work together to find an approach that suits you".

A specific model you may find useful for breaking bad news is the SPIKES model (Baile *et al.*, 2000):

SPIKES
- S: SETTING UP the interview
- P: Assessing the patient's PERCEPTION
- I: Obtaining the patient's INVITATION
- K: Giving KNOWLEDGE and information to the patient
- E: Addressing the patient's EMOTIONS with empathy
- S: STRATEGY and SUMMARY

You may be familiar with the SPIKES model from medical school. The paper by Baile and colleagues provides valuable suggestions for each stage of the model.

This book contains several practice stations, including three mock patient consultations for the "online" interview, plus three mock communication stations for the "in-person" interview format. You could consider using further practice stations for medical school finals, GP ST1 interviews and/or MRCP PACES, although the latter two may feature lengthier stations, probably involving more advanced general medical knowledge. You can also make your own mock stations to practise with a partner or group.

Useful resources for communication skills:

- Kurtz S, Silverman J, Benson J, Draper J. Marrying content and process in clinical method teaching: enhancing the Calgary–Cambridge guides. *Acad Med*. 2003;78(8):802–9.
- Baile WF, *et al.* (2000), SPIKES — A six-step protocol for delivering bad news: application to the patient with cancer. *The Oncologist*. 5:302–11.
- Consider MRCP PACES book(s).
- Consider clinical communication skills book(s).

Clinical Knowledge

For the "in-person" interview format, an entire station was traditionally dedicated to testing clinical knowledge. It is currently unclear if this format will be brought back in the future. In many ways, the clinical knowledge station was the most unpredictable because such a broad range of material could come up. Ample time is required to cover a broad range of material in preparation for this station. For the 2021 online interview format, at the time of writing, it is unclear how much clinical knowledge will be tested. A sensible approach could be to thoroughly prepare your clinical knowledge to a high standard, in case this is required for the online patient consultation. This preparation should not go to waste, as the knowledge gained should benefit you as you progress in your career.

The online patient consultation, or "in-person" clinical knowledge station, may feature an ocular manifestation of a systemic disease or a common ophthalmic condition, but anything eye-related could potentially come up. The OST1 2020 "in-person" interview guidance advises that the questions may revolve around identifying clinical signs or interpreting investigations (Severn PGME, 2020b).

A safe strategy could be to list conditions with ocular manifestations, including clinical signs and associated investigations, then read around these systematically to enhance your knowledge. Important eye conditions from reputable books and online resources could be added to this. It is difficult to provide a comprehensive list as the interview topics are all down to the discretion of the powers that be. Once again, "excess" preparation will not go to waste, as the material you learn will stand you in good stead for commencing ST1 and doing your FRCOphth exams.

Do whatever it takes to cement this knowledge in your mind, e.g., short notes, flashcards, PowerPoint slides, spider diagrams, teaching sessions with colleagues, and most importantly, mock interview practice. The three mock online patient consultations in this book feature clinical knowledge, plus three mock clinical stations are included in the three "in-person" mock interview circuits. You can make your own mock interviews too, and test yourself or a partner using as much material as possible. The more effort you put into preparation, the greater your chances of scoring highly and the lower your chances of getting caught out.

Useful resources for clinical knowledge:

- Wilkinson IB, *et al. Oxford Handbook of Clinical Medicine*. Oxford University Press; 2017.
  o Targeted reading: conditions with ocular manifestations
- Denniston AKO, Murray PI. *Oxford Handbook of Ophthalmology*. Oxford University Press; 2018.
  o Targeted reading
- Eyewiki.aao.org

Chapter **6**

Mock Online Patient Consultations

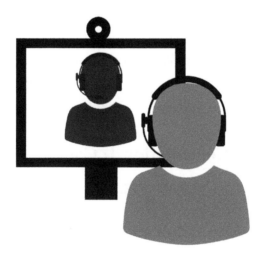

Please note: *Due to the COVID-19 pandemic, the 2021 OST interviews will be delivered virtually via Microsoft Teams. At the time of writing, it is unclear whether this will be a long-term format or whether the interviews will revert to the traditional "in-person" format in the future. Hence, this book contains chapters for both formats, with a degree of overlap between the two. Please ensure that you check the latest requirements via the Royal College of Ophthalmologists website (RCOphth, 2020a).*

This chapter contains three mock patient consultations with briefs for candidates and patients, suggested solutions and positive/ negative indicators. These are purely intended to aid your preparation and may not be fully reflective of the real online mock interviews, as these are unprecedented with limited guidance available at the time of writing. Hence, no attempt has been made to replicate the online interview stations and any similarities have arisen unintentionally. These mock stations contain a challenging mix of communication skills and clinical knowledge to give you a starting point in your preparation. You could consider using Microsoft Teams with a willing partner to mimic the online format. *Please note — the updated 2021 OST guidance advises that candidates have 3 minutes for preparation and 7 minutes for the consultation with the actor. The following three mock stations within this book are longer and more in-depth, but should still serve as useful general practice for communication skills and clinical knowledge.*

Mock Patient Consultation 1: Candidate Brief

You are an ST1 in Ophthalmology working in the diabetic retinopathy clinic. Mr John Smith is a 53-year-old male patient with poorly controlled type 2 diabetes. His chief complaint is a reduction in the central vision of his right eye. Optical coherence tomography (OCT) of the left macula was unremarkable, but OCT of the right macula has revealed diabetic macular oedema, hence he must be commenced on a series of intravitreal anti-vascular endothelial growth factor (anti-VEGF) injections in the right eye. Please conduct a consultation with Mr Smith.

Mock Patient Consultation 2: Candidate Brief

You are an ST1 in Ophthalmology, working in the Eye Casualty (Eye Emergency Department). Mrs Aisha Musa, a 65-year-old female patient with a two-day history of loss of vision in her left eye is sent to you by her optician. Her left fundus photograph shows a pale retina with a central cherry red spot, whereas her right fundus photograph is unremarkable. Hence, she has left central retinal artery occlusion (CRAO). You discuss with your consultant, who advises, due to late presentation, no treatment for CRAO is appropriate, and the patient will not regain vision in her left eye. Please conduct a consultation with Mrs Musa.

Mock Patient Consultation 3: Candidate Brief

You are an ST1 in Ophthalmology attending a cataract surgery list. Ms Lilian Fan is a 70-year-old female patient due to undergo cataract surgery today for her right eye. However, she has marked bilateral blepharitis, and you must therefore cancel her operation and reschedule it to a later date. Please conduct a consultation with Ms Fan.

Mock Patient Consultation 1: Patient Brief and Solutions

Name, gender, age, DOB:
Mr John Smith, male, 53 years old, 15 August 1967

PC:
Reduced vision — right eye

HPC:
Four-week history of gradual, painless reduction of central vision in right eye with worsening distortion (metamorphopsia). White eyes.
No other ocular symptoms:

- No flashes or floaters
- No haloes
- No peripheral visual field loss or "curtain" effect
- No redness or discharge

No new systemic symptoms:

- No headache
- No aura
- No scalp tenderness
- No jaw claudication
- No fatigue/malaise
- No nausea/vomiting/diarrhoea
- No dizziness/confusion/fainting
- No polyuria, polydipsia or polyphagia

PMH:
Type 2 diabetes mellitus (15 years), obesity, hypertension, hyper-cholesterolaemia, presbyopia (wears reading glasses).

DH:
Metformin, gliclazide, ramipril, simvastatin.

Allergies:
None known.

SH:
Smoker: half pack per day for the past 30 years; alcohol: 6 units per week ("a few pints of beer on a Friday"); lives alone, neighbour brings him to appointments; office worker for an insurance company, works full-time from home since COVID-19 pandemic/lockdown; largely sedentary lifestyle, more so since COVID-19 pandemic/lockdown, no regular exercise. Drives a car.

FH:
Father and uncle had diabetes too. Father died of a heart attack. Uncle died of a stroke.

ICE:

Provided below with corresponding suggestions for candidates (please note that these are not exhaustive).

Ideas:

- Knows that diabetes means too much sugar in the blood, but is unsure why this is a problem.
  - Candidates should explain diabetes in lay terms, e.g., diabetes is a lifelong condition that causes the blood sugar levels to become too high, which can lead to problems affecting the heart, eyes, nerves, kidneys and other organs. Normally, an organ called the pancreas makes a hormone called insulin, which the body uses to get glucose, a sugar, from food and uses this for energy. In type 2 diabetes mellitus, the body either does not produce enough insulin or resists the effects of insulin. Improving blood sugar control can reduce the risk of long-term complications.
  - Candidates could suggest providing the patient with an information leaflet for diabetes and/or diabetic retinopathy.
- Knows that his medications are for diabetes, but is unsure how they work. Suboptimal adherence to medication — he thinks that the medications should work even if he misses some days of the week.
  - Candidates should explain how metformin and gliclazide work in lay terms, e.g., metformin belongs to a class of antidiabetic medications called biguanides and works by reducing the amount of sugar that the liver releases in the blood. Gliclazide belongs to a class of antidiabetic medications called sulfonylureas and works by increasing the amount of insulin the pancreas makes, which lowers the blood sugar.

      o Candidates should emphasise the importance of strict adherence to these medications as prescribed to optimise control of blood sugar and reduce the risk of complications.

      o Candidates could explore what information and support the patient has to improve diabetic control, such as their GP, diabetes specialist nurse and DESMOND group (Diabetes Education and Self Management for Ongoing and Newly Diagnosed).

- Knows that diabetes mellitus causes diabetic retinopathy, but is unsure why.
  - o Candidates should explain diabetic retinopathy in lay terms, e.g. the retina is a structure at the back of the eye responsible for vision by converting light into electrical signals for the brain. The retina is supplied by small blood vessels. High blood sugar levels due to diabetes can damage these blood vessels, causing diabetic retinopathy. The area in the centre of the retina responsible for fine vision is called the macula. Diabetic macular oedema happens when fluid from damaged blood vessels leaks into the macula.

- Is unsure how anti-VEGF injections work.
  - o Candidates should explain VEGF and anti-VEGF in lay terms, e.g. VEGF stands for "vascular endothelial growth factor". This stimulates the formation of blood vessels. In diabetic retinopathy, too much VEGF is released in the eye, which causes abnormal blood vessels to grow and leak in the macula. This can be treated using anti-VEGF injections, which can reduce the levels of VEGF, stop the growth of abnormal new blood vessels and reduce the fluid leakage in the macula.

- Is unsure what his GP meant by "HbA1c".

- o Candidates should offer a clear explanation, e.g., HbA1c is known as glycated haemoglobin — red blood cells bonded to sugar. Red blood cells are active for 2–3 months. Therefore, HbA1c represents a person's average blood sugar levels for the last 2–3 months. A high HbA1c means that this person's blood sugar levels are too high. An ideal HbA1c level for patients with diabetes mellitus is 6.5% or below.
- Thinks he can continue to drive without informing the Driver and Vehicle Licensing Agency (DVLA) of his diabetic macular oedema that requires anti-VEGF injections.
  - o Candidates should explain that it is the patient's legal responsibility to inform the DVLA that he has diabetic retinopathy requiring injections. If he does not meet the legal eyesight standard for driving, then he should not drive.

Concerns:

- Worried that the injection will hurt.
  - o Candidates should explain that efforts are made to reduce discomfort during the intravitreal injection (e.g. numbing drops, clear explanations from staff, relaxation techniques, positioning with pillow for head and/or thighs), but the patient may still feel pressure.
- Worried that the injection might make him go blind.
  - o Candidates should explain that the injections only carry a small risk to vision and this is unusual. However, the risk to vision is far greater if patients do not receive any treatment, in which case the diabetic macular oedema could get even worse and cause permanent vision loss if left untreated.
  - o Candidates could explain that they will get an idea of whether the treatment is working by monitoring the patient's

vision and 3D scans of the retina (OCT) to check whether the diabetic macular oedema/swelling/fluid is resolving.

Expectations:

- Thinks he only needs medications on some days of the week.
  - o Candidates should emphasise the importance of strict adherence to prescribed medications in order to optimise control of blood sugar and reduce the risk of complications.
- Expects only one injection might be needed to make his vision better.
  - o Candidates should clarify that a series of injections is typically required with regular monitoring for a longer-term benefit.

Mock Patient Consultation 2: Patient Brief and Solutions

Name, gender, age, DOB:
Mrs Aisha Musa, female, 65 years old, 10 October 1955.

PC:
Loss of vision — left eye

HPC:
Sudden, painless loss of vision two days ago in her left eye. This has happened to her previously, but recovered shortly afterwards. White eyes.
No other ocular symptoms:

- No flashes or floaters

- No haloes
- No peripheral visual field loss or "curtain" effect
- No redness or discharge

No new systemic symptoms:

- No headache
- No aura
- No scalp tenderness
- No jaw claudication
- No fatigue/malaise
- No nausea/vomiting/diarrhoea
- No dizziness/confusion/fainting

PMH:
Atrial fibrillation (AF), hypertension, hypercholesterolaemia, presbyopia (wears reading glasses), one transient ischaemic attack (TIA) two years ago.

DH:
Rivaroxaban, amlodipine, candesartan, atorvastatin.

Allergies:
Penicillin.

SH:
Lives with and cares for her husband, who is unwell with lung cancer. Does not drink alcohol. Has never smoked. Works as a cleaner. Takes bus to work. Work is fairly active but no additional exercise. Does not drive a car.

FH:
Mother died of a stroke. Father died of a heart attack.

ICE:

Provided below with corresponding suggestions for candidates (please note that these are not exhaustive).

Ideas:

- Is unsure what "central retinal artery occlusion" means.
  - o Candidates must "break bad news" here. The patient may become emotional and start sobbing. One approach is to use the SPIKES framework as part of the overall consultation:
    - STEP 1: SETTING UP the interview
    - STEP 2: Assessing the patient's PERCEPTION
    - STEP 3: Obtaining the patient's INVITATION
    - STEP 4: Giving KNOWLEDGE and information to the patient
    - STEP 5: Addressing the patient's EMOTIONS with empathic responses
    - STEP 6: Strategy and summary
  - o Candidates must explain CRAO in lay terms, e.g. the retina is a structure at the back of the eye responsible for vision by converting light into electrical signals for the brain. The main blood vessel supplying the retina is the central retinal artery. A blockage of the central retinal artery is called central retinal artery occlusion.
- Is unsure why she has lost vision in her left eye, but thinks it may soon return spontaneously.
  - o The candidate should sensitively approach this subject, e.g. within the SPIKES framework, and also clarify that it is highly unlikely that vision would return to her left eye at this stage.
- Thinks that her rivaroxaban is to help her conditions, but is unsure how it actually works.

- o Candidates should explain in lay terms, e.g.,
  - Rivaroxaban is an anticoagulant or "blood thinner" used to make blood flow through the veins more easily and reduce the risk of dangerous blood clots. It works by stopping a blood-clotting factor called factor Xa. This has been prescribed because the patient has atrial fibrillation and a history of TIA, or "mini-stroke", to prevent the risk of future TIA or a stroke.

Concerns:

- She is the sole carer of her husband, who is unwell with lung cancer.
  - o Candidates should gently approach this issue, demonstrating empathy. They could use the "RAV" model:
    - Recognise that a patient has an emotional response to a situation, detecting their verbal and nonverbal cues.
    - Acknowledge this emotional response.
    - Validate their emotional response with empathy.
- She is worried about her own risk of a stroke.
  - o Candidates should express the urgent need for a same-day medical workup to reduce her risk of a stroke.
  - o Candidates could also use the RAV model here. Candidates should reiterate the importance of optimal control of risk factors to prevent a stroke with medication and lifestyle advice.

Expectations:

- She thinks that an operation can bring back the vision in her left eye if her vision does not soon return spontaneously.

o As above, candidates should gently refute this and explain that the focus should be on preserving vision in her right eye and reducing the risk of a stroke.

Mock Patient Consultation 3: Patient Brief and Solutions

Name, gender, age, DOB:

Ms Lilian Fan, female, 70 years old, 1 December 1950.

PC:

Cataract — right eye

HPC:

Six-month history of blurred vision in right eye, gradually worsening, glare, reduced ability to discern colours. In addition, a six-week history of bilateral eyelid crusting and sticking with intermittent redness and irritation.

No other ocular symptoms:

- No flashes or floaters
- No haloes
- No peripheral visual field loss or "curtain" effect

No new systemic symptoms:

- No headache
- No aura
- No scalp tenderness
- No jaw claudication
- No fever
- No fatigue/malaise
- No nausea/vomiting/diarrhoea
- No dizziness/confusion/fainting

PMH:

Hypertension, presbyopia (wears reading glasses).

DH:

Amlodipine.

Allergies:

Elastoplast.

SH:

Lives with her husband, a retired interior designer, in a ground-floor flat. Never smoked. Drinks two glasses of wine per week. Used to go for walks regularly but has been less confident since her vision deteriorated. Does not drive. Son brings them food and shopping as her husband does not drive.

FH:

Thinks her father had glaucoma — he had an operation and was using drops.

ICE:

Provided below with corresponding suggestions for candidates (please note that these are not exhaustive).

Ideas:

- Thinks she is having her cataract surgery today. Very keen as she has been waiting for three months.
  - o The candidate must "break bad news" here. One approach is to use the SPIKES framework as part of the overall consultation:
    - · STEP 1: SETTING UP the interview
    - · STEP 2: Assessing the patient's PERCEPTION

- STEP 3: Obtaining the patient's INVITATION
- STEP 4: Giving KNOWLEDGE and information to the patient
- STEP 5: Addressing the patient's EMOTIONS with empathic responses
- STEP 6: Strategy and Summary

- Is unsure why her operation must be cancelled due to blepharitis.
  o This could be included within Step 4 of the SPIKES framework, if used.
  o Candidates should explain what blepharitis is in lay terms, e.g., "Blepharitis is a common condition that causes the eyelids to become red, swollen and inflamed".
  o Candidates should explain that untreated blepharitis can increase the risk of complications following cataract surgery, including dry eyes and an increased risk of infection, including endophthalmitis — a rare but devastating infection in the eye that can cause blindness. Therefore it is important to treat blepharitis prior to cataract surgery.
- Is unsure how blepharitis can be managed.
  o Candidates should demonstrate a basic understanding of the principles in managing blepharitis with eyelid hygiene, including warm compresses, eyelid massage and/or eyelid scrubs. Topical and/or oral antibiotics are also reasonable suggestions, given the limited clinical information.
- Thinks that a cataract is a skin growing over her eye.
  o Candidates should gently refute this and explain what a cataract is in lay terms, e.g., like a camera, the eye has a lens that focuses light in the eye. If the camera lens is cloudy, it is difficult to see through a camera. Similarly, if the lens in the eye becomes cloudy, this can reduce vision. A cataract reduces the transparency of the lens, which commonly occurs with

advancing age. This can be treated with surgery by removing the cloudy lens and implanting a plastic lens so that the patient can see more clearly.

Concerns:

- She is worried that if she does not have her operation now, she could go permanently blind.
  - o Candidates can reassure the patient that it is unlikely that rearranging the date of surgery would have any significant affect on the overall outcome in this case. The reduction in vision caused by cataracts is reversible in the majority of cases.
- She is concerned that it will be difficult for her son to bring her in again as he is busy with work. This was all carefully planned in advance for today.
  - o Candidates should demonstrate empathy in their response and could suggest hospital transport as a potential solution. Candidates could consider the RAV model:
    - ▪ Recognise that a patient has an emotional response to a situation, detecting their verbal and nonverbal cues.
    - ▪ Acknowledge this emotional response.
    - ▪ Validate their emotional response with empathy.

Expectations:

- She thinks that it should only take a few days for her blepharitis to clear up.
  - o Candidates should set the patient's expectations appropriately. Blepharitis is a chronic (long-term) condition that will typically require at least 4–6 weeks of treatment before it improves sufficiently to proceed with cataract surgery.

Positive and Negative Indicators

These are simply suggestions to aid preparation/feedback for the mock online patient consultations:

Positive indicators:
- Demonstration of effective communication skills and good clinical knowledge to access relevant information in the patient brief.
- Logical flow to patient consultation.
- Clear spoken English.
- Effective use of open and closed questions.
- Delivery of medical information in plain English at an appropriate pace for the patient, checking their understanding.
- Effective exploration of ideas, concerns and expectations.
- Demonstration of empathy.

Negative indicators:
- Inability to access relevant information in the patient brief, due to poor communication skills and/or poor clinical knowledge.
- Disorganised and illogical approach to patient consultation.
- Poor spoken English.
- Poor questioning style.
- Poor delivery of medical information with too much jargon without explanation, overwhelming the patient with information, failing to check their understanding.
- Failure to explore one or more of ideas, concerns and expectations.
- No demonstration of empathy and/or impolite.

Chapter 7 The In-Person Interview

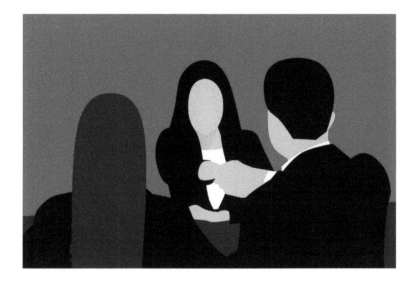

Please note: Due to the COVID-19 pandemic, the 2021 OST interviews will be delivered virtually via Microsoft Teams. At the time of writing, it is unclear whether this will be a long-term format or whether the interviews will revert to the traditional "in-person" format in the future. Hence, this book contains chapters for both formats, with a degree of overlap between the two. Please ensure you check the latest requirements via the Royal College of Ophthalmologists website (RCOphth, 2020a).

This chapter will walk you through each step of the in-person interview process in accordance with the previous guidance for 2020 in-person interviews (Severn PGME, 2020b) and provide strategies to help you score as highly as possible.

General Information

Ophthalmology ST1 interviews have been centralised since 2012. The interviews are co-ordinated by the Severn Deanery and are usually held in February in a hotel in Bristol. Travel expenses can be claimed via Selenity according to the national expenses policy (HEE, 2020). If you live far away, it may be worth staying in a nearby hotel to ensure you arrive on time. The Severn Deanery advises that candidates requiring accommodation must not stay at the hotel where the interviews are held.

When you arrive, you should report to the reception for registration and ID checks — you will already have received information for what is required at this stage. You can leave coats and non-valuable luggage in the cloakroom. The whole process may take up to three hours, so bring food and drink or be prepared to buy these onsite or nearby.

Be sure to plan your outfit. You should wear a professional outfit that makes you feel confident. Consider a toilet break and a quick mirror check before your interview to check whether you are presentable. Take deep breaths and remain cool, calm and collected. You are highly capable, and this is your time to shine.

Structure

The following table provides an outline of the interview structure following registration, including timing and scoring as per the OST1 2020 interview guidance (Severn PGME, 2020b):

Outline of OST1 Interview Structure

Task	Description	Max. Score	Time
Preparation	Scenarios and paper to review	N/A	40 mins
Portfolio Review	Portfolio is assessed by two panel members alongside interview stations	100	20 mins
Station A	Critical appraisal (8 mins)	30	16 mins
	Improving patient care (8 mins)	40	
Station B	Communication scenario (7 mins)	40	16 mins
	Clinical knowledge (9 mins)	50	

Preparation stage

Following registration, you will be taken to the preparation room and briefed on the preparation and interview process. After this, the 40-minute countdown will begin and you will review a published paper and read different scenarios, including improving patient care and patient history for the communication scenario. Typically, clinical knowledge may involve reviewing images/videos on an iPad.

Once you become well practised, you will see the 40-minute preparation stage as a gift. This is a golden opportunity to consolidate your thoughts and plan efficiently for the stations. This should be rehearsed strictly to time during your interview practice, as this will help you optimise your performance under time pressure.

Scoring and offers

According to the previous guidance for the 2020 in-person interviews (Severn PGME, 2020b), there are 160 points in total across the in-person interview stations A and B. This is added to the portfolio score (max. 100) and MSRA (max. 40) to bring the total possible score to 300.

Once the interviews have taken place, all candidates will be ranked in order of their total scores. Available OST1 posts will be allocated according to ranking. Any candidates who fail to achieve a minimum score of 180/300 (60%) or a minimum score in two or more questions within the interview stations (12/30; 16/40; 20/50; i.e., 40%) will be excluded from the ranking and offers process.

Critical Appraisal

Critical appraisal is the process of systematically assessing the validity and relevance of research in a particular setting. This is a highly important skill for all doctors to attain. The art of critical appraisal is a subject unto itself, requiring specialised texts and resources beyond the scope of this book. Nonetheless, a broad overview is provided along with three practice critical appraisal stations in the mock interviews chapter.

A good standard of critical appraisal is expected in the OST1 interview. Ideally, you should keep training until you can pick up an unfamiliar paper, read it in a relatively short time, understand its nuts and bolts and be able to discuss its strengths and weaknesses with confidence and fluency. You are fully capable of achieving this, but it will not happen overnight. For the OST1 interview, I would recommend a specialised book and online resources to learn the art of critical appraisal and practise, practise, practise.

Thorough preparation could enable you to score full marks or thereabouts on this station.

Despite being worth fewer marks compared to the other stations, reviewing the paper and making notes to answer the questions will likely take up the majority of your 40 minutes of preparation time. However, this is worth it as the marks are highly achievable. As a general rule, aim to complete this preparation in no more than 25 minutes.

The Critical Appraisal Skills Programme (CASP, 2020) checklists are helpful for developing a systematic approach to critically appraising a paper. Note that there are checklists for eight types of study:

1. Systematic review
2. Qualitative
3. Randomised controlled trial (RCT)
4. Case-control
5. Diagnostic
6. Cohort
7. Economic evaluation
8. Clinical prediction rule

Don't be tempted to only focus on RCTs. You could be given any paper to critically appraise, so the safe approach would be to cover all bases by preparing for all study types, albeit it is unlikely that you would receive types 7 or 8.

The questions about the paper could involve any part of the critical appraisal process. You should become fluent in discussing internal and external validity including all types of bias. Internal validity relates to how well a study is conducted, while external validity relates to how generalisable the findings are to other groups and settings. You must also become *au fait* with statistical testing and terminology.

For practice, you can search for open access papers online (or papers that you can access via an institutional account). It is one thing to be able to read and understand a scientific paper, but another thing altogether to complete this interview task under time pressure. Therefore, it would be wise to regularly practise critically appraising papers in no more than 25 minutes. Practise, practise, practise — I cannot emphasise this enough. Ultimately, success in this station (and all stations) will be achieved by those who want it the most.

Useful resources for critical appraisal:

- Gosall NK, Gosall GS. *The Doctor's Guide to Critical Appraisal.* Pastest; 2020.
- Greenhalgh T. *How to Read a Paper: The Basics of Evidence-based Medicine and Healthcare.* Wiley-Blackwell; 2019.
- Papers (institutional/open access).

Improving Patient Care

This station tests your understanding of clinical audit and quality improvement (QI) projects. First, we must define these terms.

This is the definition for clinical audit endorsed by the National Institute for Health and Care Excellence (NICE, 2002):

"Clinical audit is a (quality improvement) process that seeks to improve patient care and outcomes through systematic review of care against explicit criteria and the implementation of change."

I have bracketed "quality improvement" in the above definition as it perhaps confuses matters using this specific term when defining clinical audit. The above definition for clinical audit was published in 2002, whereas the role and popularity of QI has grown more recently.

Here is a definition for QI by Batalden and Davidoff (2007):

"The combined and unceasing efforts of everyone — healthcare professionals, patients and their families, researchers, payers, planners and educators — to make the changes that will lead to better patient outcomes (health), better system performance (care) and better professional development."

There is a key difference between these two definitions — established standards. A clinical audit asks the question "how are we performing?" against established standards, while QI projects ask: "How do we actually improve?" While an audit assumes conditional stability, QI involves continual improvement in unstable conditions. To improve your understanding of both, find examples of clinical audits and QI projects in the published literature and your local setting. Be aware that not everyone uses these terms correctly. Moreover, there can be a degree of crossover between audit, QI and research.

With respect to QI, the US Institute of Medicine has defined six dimensions of quality in healthcare (Institute of Medicine, 1990):

1. *Safe* — avoiding harm to patients from care that is intended to help them.
2. *Effective* — providing evidence-based services that produce a clear benefit.
3. *Patient-centred* — providing care that is responsive to and respectful of the patient's needs and values.
4. *Timely* — reducing waits and sometimes harmful delays.
5. *Efficient* — avoiding waste.
6. *Equitable* — providing care that does not vary based on a patient's personal characteristics.

You can remember these with the acronym "SEPTEE". Another important acronym to know relates to the goals for either a clinical audit or QI project. These goals should be "SMART" (Yemm, 2013):

- Specific
- Measurable
- Achievable
- Relevant
- Time-bound

There are a number of variations on what the letters stand for depending on the source you use, such as "A" for "Assignable" or "R" for "Realistic". Some extend this to "SMARTER", adding "Evaluated" and "Reviewed". The point of the SMART approach is to carefully consider the "who", "what", "where", "when", "why" and "how".

There are different ways of expressing the stages involved in the clinical audit cycle. Five stages are recommended by NICE (2002):

The Clinical Audit Cycle

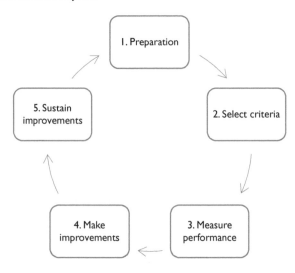

These five stages address the following five questions:

1. What are we trying to achieve?
2. Are we achieving it?
3. Why are we not achieving it?
4. What can we do to make things better?
5. Have we made things better?

You should also be familiar with the PDSA (Plan-Do-Study-Act) cycle (Gillam and Siriwardena, 2013), summarised in the figure below:

The PDSA Cycle

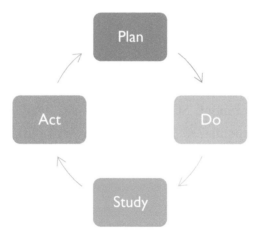

This model can be applied to QI (and to audit too, broadly speaking). First, a plan must be developed with a clear objective (*Plan*). Next, the plan should be executed and data collected (*Do*). This data should be analysed (*Study*). Finally, appropriate changes can be introduced to improve outcomes (*Act*). There are specific SQUIRE (2017) guidelines for reporting quality improvement projects.

It is crucial to involve and actively engage **key stakeholders** throughout your audit or QI project from the very beginning. In this context, key stakeholders are parties who can affect or be affected by your project. This could include healthcare professionals of various backgrounds, managers, administrative staff, IT staff, clinical coders, related organisations, charities, patients and members of the public. This list is not exhaustive. NHS Improvement has produced in-depth information and tools to facilitate stakeholder analysis (NHS Improvement, 2018).

Useful resources for audit/QI:

- RCR. Quality improvement. https://www.rcr.ac.uk/clinical-radiology/audit-and-qi/quality-improvement. Accessed Sept 2020.
- RCR. Audit and quality improvement. https://www.rcr.ac.uk/clinical-radiology/audit-and-quality-improvement. Accessed Sept 2020.
- NHS Improvement. Stakeholder analysis. https://improvement.nhs.uk/documents/2169/stakeholder-analysis.pdf. Accessed Sept 2020.

8 Mock In-Person Interview Circuits

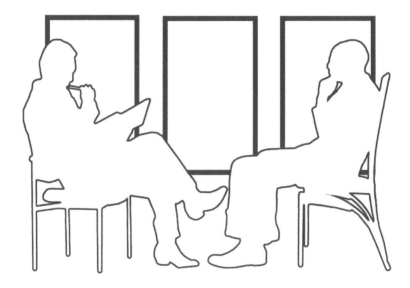

Please note: All of the included mock interview circuits have been developed by the author. These are not official OST1 interview questions or solutions — they are simply designed to help enhance your knowledge and prepare good interview technique under timed conditions. No attempts have been made to replicate previous OST1 interview scenarios. Any similarities to previous or future OST1 interview scenarios have arisen unintentionally and by chance.

This section contains three mock interview circuits. Spend your allotted 40 minutes of preparation time reviewing all material except the clinical knowledge questions. Then, answer the questions with a volunteer examiner, strictly adhering to the time limits. Consider video recording your performances so you can reflect on your answers and body language. Your examiner can refer to the solutions in the next chapter while interviewing you.

9 Circuit 1: Questions

Circuit 1: Critical Appraisal

Review the following paper available online:

> Lehman CD, Wellman RD, Buist DSM, *et al*. Diagnostic accuracy of digital screening mammography with and without computer-aided detection. *JAMA Intern Med*. 2015; 175(11):1828–37. doi:10.1001/jamainternmed.2015.5231

1. Summarise the study methodology.
2. Give three potential sources of bias in this study and how they were minimised.
3. Define sensitivity and specificity.
4. List five World Health Organization criteria for screening tests.

Circuit 1: Improving Patient Care

You are an FY2 working in the acute medical unit (AMU). You notice that some of your colleagues do not always complete the venous thromboembolism (VTE) risk assessment form in a timely fashion. You are aware that the NHS target for VTE risk assessment on admission is 95%. You decide to conduct an audit for VTE risk assessment in your AMU.

1. How would you plan and conduct this audit?
2. Who would you involve in your audit?

3. How could you promote best practice in light of your audit findings?
4. What is the difference between an audit and a quality improvement project?

Circuit 1: Communication Scenario

You are the Ophthalmology ST1 working in the medical retina clinic. Your patient is a 70-year-old lady with advanced age-related macular degeneration (AMD). Her vision has deteriorated to such an extent that no further treatment is possible, and she now meets the criteria to be registered as severely sight impaired (blind). Please proceed to the consultation room to speak with the patient.

Your examiner should refer to the corresponding briefing notes in the Mock In-Person Interview Solutions chapter.

Circuit 1: Clinical Knowledge Part A

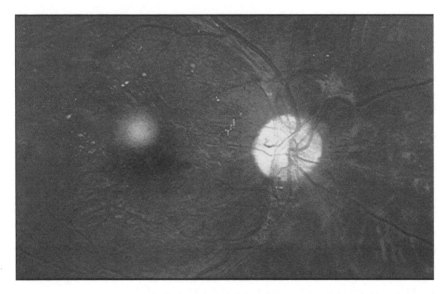

Image credit: Mr Hussein Almuhtaseb, Consultant Ophthalmic Surgeon, Bradford Royal Infirmary, UK

1. Which pathological sign in this fundus photograph poses the greatest threat to vision?
2. Which signalling protein is responsible for the development of this pathology?
3. List four symptoms of diabetes mellitus.
4. List four chronic complications of diabetes mellitus.
5. Name a landmark trial for the treatment of diabetic retinopathy.

Circuit 1: Clinical Knowledge Part B

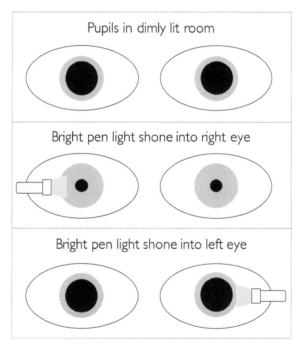

6. What pathological sign is depicted in this figure?
7. List three causes for this pathological sign.
8. Which cranial nerve carries the afferent limb involved in the pupillary light reflex?
9. What name is given to a pupil that accommodates but does not react to light?

Circuit 1: Clinical Knowledge Part C

A 50-year-old gentleman presents to the clinic with the following Humphrey visual field test result:

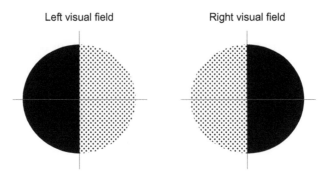

Left visual field   Right visual field

10. What visual field defect is displayed above?
11. Where is the lesion located?
12. Name three potential causes of this visual field defect.
13. This gentleman has prominent supraorbital ridges, jaw enlargement and hirsutism. Name two systemic complications commonly associated with this condition.
14. This gentleman complains that distant objects seem to vanish when he looks at near objects. What term is used to describe this phenomenon?

10 Circuit 2: Questions

Circuit 2: Critical Appraisal

Review the following paper available online:

> Gazzard G, Konstantakopoulou E, Garway-Heath D, *et al*. Selective laser trabeculoplasty versus eye drops for first-line treatment of ocular hypertension and glaucoma (LiGHT): a multicentre randomised controlled trial. *Lancet*. 2019; 393(10180):1505–16. doi:10.1016/ S0140-6736(18)32213-X

1. Summarise the findings and implications of this study.
2. Give four strengths of this study.
3. Give four weaknesses of this study.
4. Define what is meant by a 95% confidence interval.
5. What is an intention to treat analysis?

Circuit 2: Improving Patient Care

You are an ST1 working in a glaucoma clinic that frequently runs late. There has been an increase in the number of patients complaining about the long waiting times. You decide to conduct a quality improvement project to address the long waiting times for this clinic.

1. How would you plan and conduct this quality improvement project?

2. Who would you involve in your quality improvement project?
3. What actions would you take after completing this quality improvement project?
4. What is the difference between a quality improvement project and an audit?

Circuit 2: Communication Scenario

You are the Ophthalmology ST1 assisting a cataract theatre list. The time is 16:30. Your consultant has just accepted an emergency procedure from the on-call registrar. Your consultant has therefore asked you to inform the final patient awaiting cataract surgery that their procedure must be cancelled and postponed to a later date. The final patient, an 80-year-old gentleman, has been asked to wait in the consultation room for you. Please proceed to the consultation room to speak with the patient.

Your examiner should refer to the corresponding briefing notes in the Mock In-Person Interview Solutions chapter.

Circuit 2: Clinical Knowledge Part A

Please read this optician's referral to the Eye Casualty (Eye Emergency Department):

Crystal View Opticians

Dear Eye Casualty Doctor,

Re: Mr Albert Fisher; DOB: 05/07/1953; Hosp. No. 12345678
This gentleman has presented with a 1-hour history of sudden loss of vision in the left eye. He has a history of hypertension and stroke. On fundoscopy, right fundus is unremarkable, while left retina is pale with a cherry-red spot in the centre. Please see him urgently. Many thanks.

---

1. What is the most likely diagnosis?
2. List five risk factors associated with this pathology.

Circuit 2: Clinical Knowledge Part B

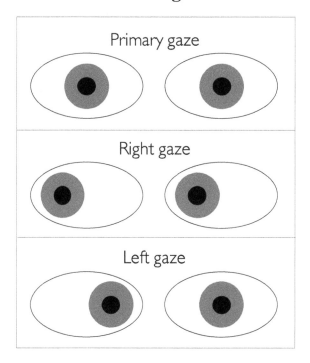

3. What pathology are these eye movements consistent with?
4. List four possible causes for this pathology in adults.
5. List four risk factors for the development of this pathology in adults.

Circuit 2: Clinical Knowledge Part C

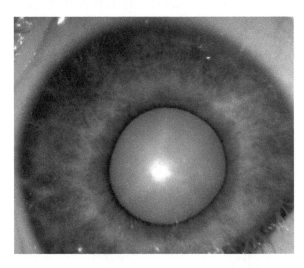

Image credit: Prof. I Christopher Lloyd, Consultant Ophthalmic Surgeon, Great Ormond Street Hospital for Children, UK

6. What is the main condition shown in this image?
7. List four symptoms that patients commonly experience with this condition.
8. List four risk factors for the development of this condition.
9. Would this patient's condition cause a relative afferent pupillary defect (RAPD)?

11 Circuit 3: Questions

Circuit 3: Critical Appraisal

Review the following paper available online:

> Lee W, Lee S, Bae H, Kim CY, Seong GJ. Efficacy and tolerability of preservative-free 0.0015% tafluprost in glaucoma patients: a prospective crossover study. *BMC Ophthalmol.* 2017; 17(1):61. doi:10.1186/s12886-017-0453-z

1. Summarise the study methodology.
2. Give three potential sources of bias in this study and how they were minimised.
3. Explain the sample size calculation.
4. What is the difference between type I and type II errors?

Circuit 3: Improving Patient Care

You are an FY2 working on the general surgery firm. You feel that the night shift handover meeting is often rushed and unstandardised. You decide to conduct a quality improvement project for general surgery night shift handover meetings.

1. How would you plan and conduct this quality improvement project?
2. Who would you involve in your quality improvement project?
3. How would you disseminate the findings of your quality improvement project?

4. How could you ensure a long-term improvement in the quality of nightshift handover in general surgery after you leave the firm?

Circuit 3: Communication Scenario

You are the Ophthalmology ST1 working in the glaucoma clinic. Your patient is a 60-year-old gentleman newly referred from the optician, who suspects chronic open angle glaucoma with significant visual field loss. Your examination and visual field testing confirm this. You must communicate this diagnosis to the patient and inform him that he should inform the Driver and Vehicle Licensing Agency (DVLA) that he can no longer drive a vehicle. Please proceed to the consultation room to speak with the patient.

Your examiner should refer to the corresponding briefing notes in the Mock In-Person Interview Solutions chapter.

Circuit 3: Clinical Knowledge Part A

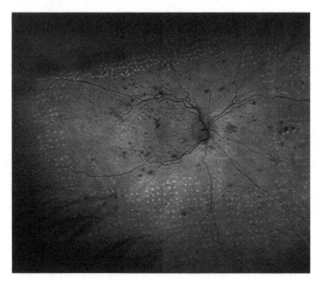

Image credit: Mr Hussein Almuhtaseb, Consultant Ophthalmic Surgeon, Bradford Royal Infirmary, UK

1. What procedure has been performed in this patient?
2. How does this procedure prevent the progression of diabetic retinopathy?
3. List three risk factors for the progression of diabetic retinopathy.
4. List three classes of oral drugs used in the treatment of diabetes mellitus.

Circuit 3: Clinical Knowledge Part B

A 35-year-old woman is referred to your ophthalmology clinic with the following blood test results:

Test	Result	Normal Range
TSH	<0.05 mU/l	0.5–5.5 mU/l
Thyroxine (T4)	196 nmol/l	70–140 nmol/l

5. List four systemic signs that this patient may display.
6. List four ocular signs that this patient may display.
7. Why might colour vision be affected in this patient?
8. Name one clinical scoring system for the severity of the eye disease commonly associated with this condition.

Circuit 3: Clinical Knowledge Part C

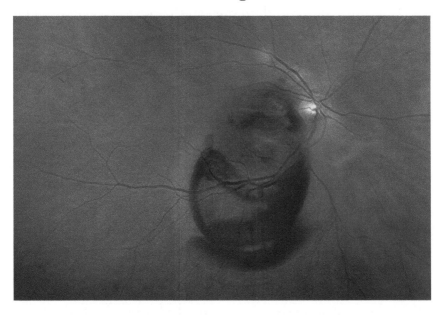

Image credit: Mr Hussein Almuhtaseb, Consultant Ophthalmic Surgeon, Bradford Royal Infirmary, UK

9. What condition is depicted in this fundus photograph?
10. Name three risk factors for the progression of this condition.
11. Which non-invasive imaging technique helps to monitor the status of this condition?
12. Name one drug used to treat this condition.
13. Name a landmark trial relating to the treatment of this condition.

12 Mock In-Person Interview Solutions

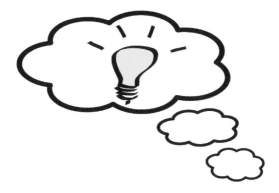

Please note: *All the included mock interview circuits have been developed by the author. These are not official OST1 interview questions or solutions — they are simply designed to help enhance your knowledge and prepare good interview technique under timed conditions. No attempts have been made to replicate previous OST1 interview scenarios. Any similarities to previous or future OST1 interview scenarios have arisen unintentionally and by chance.*

This section contains solutions for the three mock interview circuits. Rough mark schemes have been included as teaching tools, but the solutions are not strictly exhaustive. The OST interview panel ultimately decides the awarding of marks.

13 Circuit 1: Solutions

Circuit 1: Critical Appraisal

Review the following paper available online:

> Lehman CD, Wellman RD, Buist DSM, *et al.* Diagnostic accuracy of digital screening mammography with and without computer-aided detection. *JAMA Intern Med.* 2015; 175(11):1828–37. doi:10.1001/jamainternmed.2015.5231

1. Summarise the study methodology.

A coherent summary of the study methodology that demonstrates a good understanding of the study design.

2. Give three potential sources of bias in this study and how they were minimised.

Any three appropriate sources of bias presented along with how these were minimised.

3. Define sensitivity and specificity.

Sensitivity is the ability of a test to correctly identify those with the condition (true positive rate). Specificity is the ability of the test to correctly identify those without the condition (true negative rate).

   (Tip: SPIN and SNOUT: SPecific tests rule IN the condition when positive; SeNsitive tests rule OUT the condition when negative.)

4. List five World Health Organization criteria for screening tests.

Any five of the following (WHO, 2010):

- The condition should be an important health problem.
- There should be a treatment for the condition.
- Facilities for diagnosis and treatment should be available.
- There should be a latent stage of the disease.
- There should be a test for the condition.
- The test should be acceptable to the population.
- The natural history of the disease should be adequately understood.
- There should be an agreed policy on who to treat.
- The total cost of finding a case should be economically balanced in relation to medical expenditure as a whole.
- Case finding should be a continuous process, not just a "once and for all" project.
- The test used should be sensitive.

Circuit 1: Improving Patient Care

You are an FY2 working in the acute medical unit (AMU). You notice that some of your colleagues do not always complete the venous thromboembolism (VTE) risk assessment form in a timely fashion. You are aware that the NHS target for VTE risk assessment on admission is 95%. You decide to conduct an audit for VTE risk assessment in your AMU.

1. How would you plan and conduct this audit?

Good candidates will present a coherent and carefully considered plan. They should use an appropriate framework (i.e. Clinical Audit Cycle) in planning the audit and state clear objectives.

2. Who would you involve in your audit?

Good candidates will present a carefully considered strategy to ensure all key stakeholders are involved, including "who", "why", "when", "where" and "how". They will also give appropriate examples specific to the audit. They will not simply reel off a rehearsed list of MDT members.

3. How could you promote best practice in light of your audit findings?

Good candidates will present a robust post-intervention plan covering dissemination (e.g. presenting at appropriate local/ regional and national meetings, producing posters and/or digital material, publishing an audit report) as well as future directions for the project.

4. What is the difference between an audit and a quality improvement project?

Two acceptable definitions with distinctions, e.g. Clinical audit is a process that seeks to improve patient care and outcomes through a systematic review of care **against explicit criteria** and the implementation of change, assuming conditional stability,

WHEREAS

Quality improvement is a systematic approach using specific techniques, methods, measurement and strategies to continually improve one or more of the dimensions of quality healthcare (safe, effective, patient-centred, timely, efficient and equitable) involving unstable conditions.

Circuit 1: Communication Scenario

You are the Ophthalmology ST1 working in the medical retina clinic. Your patient is a 70-year-old lady with advanced age-related macular degeneration (AMD). Her vision has deteriorated to such an extent that no further treatment is possible, and she now meets the criteria to be registered as severely sight impaired (blind). Please proceed to the consultation room to speak with the patient.

Briefing notes for the patient

- You were under the impression that you could have more injections in your eye to make your sight better.
- Your friend also had advanced AMD but she got better with injections, so you thought you would too.
- You read about a special trial where they restored sight in AMD patients using stem cells — can't this be done here?
- You have just been given a paperback book that you wanted to read after your treatment.

Good candidates will employ effective communication skills to address the ideas, concerns and expectations of the patient. Effective use of open and closed questions, active listening and empathy are required to score highly. Poor candidates will not successfully access the information in the patient's briefing notes.

Circuit 1: Clinical Knowledge Part A

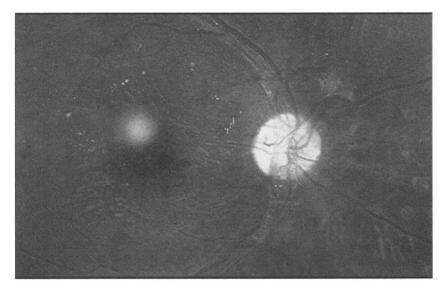

Image credit: Mr Hussein Almuhtaseb, Consultant Ophthalmic Surgeon, Bradford Royal Infirmary, UK

1. Which pathological sign in this fundus photograph poses the greatest threat to vision?

Neovascularisation of disc/new vessels on disc (2 marks)

2. Which signalling protein is responsible for the development of this pathology?

Vascular endothelial growth factor (2 marks)

3. List four symptoms of diabetes mellitus.

Any four of the following (2 marks each, 8 marks max.):

- Polyuria
- Polydipsia
- Polyphagia

- Unexplained weight loss
- Nausea and vomiting
- Fatigue
- Blurred vision
- Dry mouth
- Skin changes, including dryness, itching and acanthosis nigricans

4. List four chronic complications of diabetes mellitus.
Any four of the following (2 marks each, 8 marks max.):

- Diabetic nephropathy
- Diabetic neuropathy
- Diabetic retinopathy
- Diabetic foot syndrome
- Cardiovascular disease
- Impotence
- Skin infections

5. Name a landmark trial for the treatment of diabetic retinopathy.
Any one of the following (2 marks):

- Diabetic Retinopathy Study (DRS)[1]
- Early Treatment Diabetic Retinopathy Study (ETDRS)[2]

---

[1] Diabetic Retinopathy Study Research Group. *Am J Ophthalmology*. 1976; 81:383–96.

[2] ETDRS Research Group. *Am J Ophthalmol*. 127:137–41, 1999.

- Diabetic Retinopathy Vitrectomy Study (DRVS)[3]
- Ranibizumab (Lucentis) trials:
  - Diabetic Retinopathy Clinical Research Network (DRCR. net)[4]
  - RESOLVE[5], RESTORE[6], RISE/RIDE[7], READ-2[8]
- Bevacizumab (Avastin) trials:
  - DRCR.net[9]
  - BOLT[10]
- Aflibercept (Eylea) trials:
  - DA VINCI[11]
  - VISTA/VIVID[12]
- Any other suitable landmark trial

---

[3] The Diabetic Retinopathy Vitrectomy Study Research Group. *Arch Ophthalmol.* 1985; 103(11):1644–52.

[4] Diabetic Retinopathy Clinical Research Network. *Ophthalmology.* 2010; 117(6):1064–77.

[5] Massin P, *et al.* (RESOLVE study). *Diabetes Care.* 2010; 33(11):2399–2405.

[6] RESTORE study group. *Ophthalmology.* 2011; 118(4):615–25.

[7] Boyer DS, *et al.* (RIDE and RISE trials). *Ophthalmology.* 2015; 122(12): 2504–13.

[8] READ-2 Study Group. *Ophthalmology.* 2009; 116(11):2175–81.

[9] Diabetic Retinopathy Clinical Research Network. *Ophthalmology.* 2007; 114(10):1860–67.

[10] Michaelides M, *et al.* (BOLT study). *Ophthalmology.* 2010; 117(6):1078–86.

[11] Da Vinci Study Group. *Ophthalmology.* 2012; 119(8):1658–65.

[12] Brown DM, *et al.* (VISTA and VIVID studies). *Ophthalmology.* 2015; 122(10):2044–52.

Circuit 1: Clinical Knowledge Part B

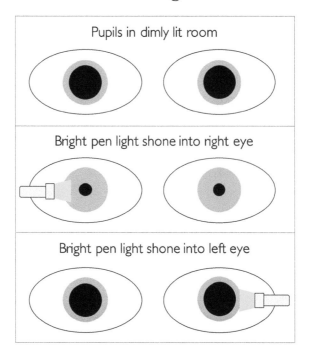

6. What pathological sign is depicted in this figure?
Left relative afferent pupillary defect / left RAPD (1 mark for stating "left", 1 mark for RAPD)

7. List three causes for this pathological sign.
Any three of the following (2 marks each, 6 marks max.):

- Ischaemic optic neuropathy
- Optic neuritis
- Optic nerve compression
- Optic nerve tumour
- Compressive optic neuropathy
- Hereditary optic neuropathy
- Trauma
- Glaucoma

- Intraocular tumour
- Ischaemic retinal disease
- Retinal infection
- Retinal detachment
- Iatrogenic

8. Which cranial nerve carries the afferent limb involved in the pupillary light reflex?

Optic nerve (2 marks)

9. What name is given to a pupil that accommodates but does not react to light?

Argyll Robertson pupil (2 marks)

Circuit 1: Clinical Knowledge Part C

A 50-year-old gentleman presents to the clinic with the following Humphrey visual field test result:

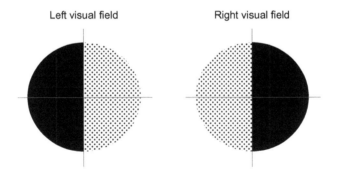

10. What visual field defect is displayed above?

Bitemporal hemianopia / bitemporal hemianopsia (2 marks)

11. Where is the lesion located?

Optic chiasm (2 marks)

12. Name three potential causes of this visual field defect.
Any three of the following (2 marks each, 6 marks max.):

- Pituitary adenoma
- Craniopharyngioma
- Rathke cleft cyst
- Suprasellar meningioma
- Internal carotid artery aneurysm

13. This gentleman has prominent supraorbital ridges, jaw enlargement and hirsutism. Name two systemic complications commonly associated with this condition.
Any two of the following (2 marks each, 4 marks max.):

- Diabetes mellitus
- Hypertension
- Congestive heart failure
- Cardiomyopathy
- Osteoarthritis
- Carpal tunnel syndrome
- Sleep apnoea

Note: These symptoms are consistent with acromegaly.

14. This gentleman complains that distant objects seem to vanish when he looks at near objects. What term is used to describe this phenomenon?
Post-fixation blindness (2 marks)
Note: This occurs due to the eyes converging on the near object, causing the impaired temporal fields to overlap. Thus, the distant object is not seen.

14 Circuit 2: Solutions

Circuit 2 Solutions: Critical Appraisal

Review the following paper available online:

> Gazzard G, Konstantakopoulou E, Garway-Heath D, *et al*. Selective laser trabeculoplasty versus eye drops for first-line treatment of ocular hypertension and glaucoma (LiGHT): a multicentre randomised controlled trial. *Lancet*. 2019; 393(10180):1505–16. doi:10.1016/S0140-6736(18)32213-X

1. Summarise the findings and implications of this study.

Good candidates will provide a coherent summary of key findings and implications with some clinical context provided in the paper. They will demonstrate an understanding of the study implications rather than simply reading off the abstract or "research in context" box.

2. Give four strengths of this study.

Any four study strengths that promote good science and reduce the risk of bias, relating to any aspect of its conduct.

3. Give four weaknesses of this study.

Any four weaknesses that affect the internal or external validity of the study and/or introduce avoidable sources of bias.

4. Define what is meant by a 95% confidence interval.

A 95% confidence interval is a range of values that you can be 95% certain contains the true mean of the population.

5. What is an intention to treat analysis?

The intention to treat (ITT) analysis includes all randomised patients in the groups to which they were randomly assigned, regardless of their adherence with the entry criteria, treatment they actually received, and subsequent withdrawal from treatment or deviation from the protocol (Fisher *et al.*, 1990). In short, "once randomised, always analysed".

Circuit 2 Solutions: Improving Patient Care

You are an ST1 working in a glaucoma clinic, which frequently runs late. There has been an increase in the number of patients complaining about the long waiting times. You decide to conduct a quality improvement project to address the long waiting times for this clinic.

1. How would you plan and conduct this quality improvement project?

Good candidates will present a coherent and carefully considered plan. They should link the problem being addressed to the appropriate dimension(s) of quality in healthcare (SEPTEE: safe, effective, patient-centred, timely, efficient and equitable). They should use an appropriate framework (i.e., PDSA) in planning the QI project and state clear objectives.

2. Who would you involve in your quality improvement project?

Good candidates will present a carefully considered strategy to ensure all key stakeholders are involved, including "who", "why", "when", "where" and "how". They will also give appropriate examples specific to the QI project. They will not simply reel off a rehearsed list of MDT members.

3. What actions would you take after completing this quality improvement project?

Good candidates will present a robust post-intervention plan covering dissemination (e.g., presenting at appropriate local/regional and national meetings, producing posters and/or digital material, publishing QI report using SQUIRE guidelines) as well as future directions for the project.

4. What is the difference between a quality improvement project and an audit?

Candidates should provide two acceptable definitions, e.g., Clinical audit is a process that seeks to improve patient care and outcomes through a systematic review of care **against explicit criteria** and the implementation of change, assuming conditional stability,

WHEREAS

Quality improvement is a systematic approach using specific techniques, methods, measurement and strategies to continually improve one or more of the dimensions of quality healthcare (safe, effective, patient-centred, timely, efficient and equitable) involving unstable conditions.

Circuit 2 Solutions: Communication Scenario

You are the Ophthalmology ST1 assisting a cataract theatre list. The time is 16:30. Your consultant has just accepted an emergency procedure from the on-call registrar. Your consultant has therefore asked you to inform the final patient awaiting cataract surgery that their procedure must be cancelled and postponed to a later date. The final patient, an 80-year-old gentleman, has been asked to wait in the consultation room for you. Please proceed to the consultation room to speak with the patient.

Briefing notes for the patient

When prompted, give the following information:

- You live alone and your daughter had difficulty getting the day off work to transport you here.
- You want to know why you were last on the list today.
- You want to know how long it will take until you will have your operation.
- You are worried that if you do not have the operation soon you could go blind because your vision keeps getting worse.

Good candidates will employ effective communication skills to address the ideas, concerns and expectations of the patient. Effective use of open and closed questions, active listening and empathy are required to score highly. Poor candidates will not successfully access the information in the patient's briefing notes.

Circuit 2: Clinical Knowledge Part A

Please read this optician's referral to the Eye Casualty (Eye Emergency Department):

Crystal View Opticians

Dear Eye Casualty Doctor,

Re: Mr Albert Fisher; DOB: 05/07/1953; Hosp. No. 12345678

This gentleman has presented with a 1-hour history of sudden loss of vision in the left eye. He has a history of hypertension and stroke. On fundoscopy, right fundus is unremarkable, while left retina is pale with a cherry-red spot in the centre. Please see him urgently. Many thanks.

---

1. What is the most likely diagnosis?
Left central retinal artery occlusion (2 marks)

2. List five risk factors associated with this pathology.
Any five of the following (2 marks each, 10 marks max.)

- Advanced age
- Male gender
- Smoking
- Obesity
- Hypertension
- Diabetes mellitus
- Cardiovascular disease
- Hypercholesterolaemia
- Coagulopathy

Circuit 2: Clinical Knowledge Part B

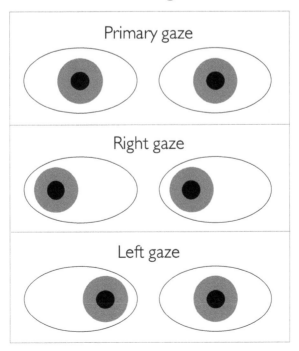

3. What pathology are these eye movements consistent with?
Sixth cranial nerve (abducens) palsy (2 marks)

4. List four possible causes for this pathology in adults.
Any four of the following (2 marks each, 8 marks max.):

- Microvascular ischaemia
- Idiopathic
- Trauma
- Giant cell arteritis
- Stroke
- Tumour
- Multiple sclerosis
- Sarcoidosis
- Vasculitis
- Intracranial hypertension

5. List four risk factors for the development of this pathology in adults.
Any four of the following (2 marks each, 8 marks max.):

- Ischaemic heart disease
- Microvascular conditions
- Smoking
- Diabetes mellitus
- Hypertension
- Hypercholesterolaemia
- Arteriosclerosis

Circuit 2: Clinical Knowledge Part C

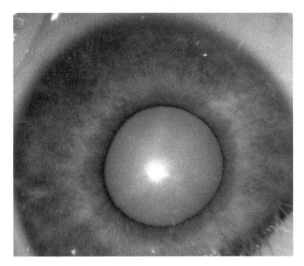

Image credit: Prof. I Christopher Lloyd, Consultant Ophthalmic Surgeon, Great Ormond Street Hospital for Children, UK

6. What is the condition shown in this image?
Cataract (2 marks)

7. List four symptoms that patients commonly experience with this condition.
Any four of the following (2 marks each, 8 marks max.):

- Reduced visual acuity
- Blurred vision
- Reduced contrast sensitivity
- Glare
- Poor night vision
- Reduced ability to distinguish between colours, or colours appear faded.
- Change in refractive status

8. List four risk factors for the development of this condition.
Any three of the following (2 marks each, 8 marks max.):

- Advancing age
- Diabetes mellitus
- Ultraviolet light exposure
- Steroid use
- Smoking
- Trauma
- Genetics
- Previous ocular surgery

9. Would this patient's condition cause a relative afferent pupillary defect (RAPD)?

No (2 marks)

Note: A cataract will not cause RAPD, provided the light is sufficiently bright and the retina and optic nerve are healthy.

15 Circuit 3: Solutions

Circuit 3: Critical Appraisal

Review the following paper available online:

> Lee W, Lee S, Bae H, Kim CY, Seong GJ. Efficacy and tolerability of preservative-free 0.0015% tafluprost in glaucoma patients: a prospective crossover study. *BMC Ophthalmol.* 2017; 17(1):61. doi:10.1186/s12886-017-0453-z

1. Summarise the study methodology.

A coherent summary of the study methodology, demonstrating a good understanding of the study design.

2. Give three potential sources of bias in this study and how they were minimised.

Any three appropriate sources of bias presented along with how these were minimised.

3. Explain the sample size calculation.

The sample size calculation determines the minimum number of participants to enrol in the study for adequate power, given certain assumptions (effect size, power, α). Adequate power reduces the risk of a type II error (non-rejection of a false null hypothesis). In this case, 20 participants were required to achieve power.

Note: It appears that the authors have confused effect size and power in their paper. In their sample size calculation, they have set power to 80%, α to 0.05, and they have not reported the effect size. Their sample size calculation may therefore be inappropriate.

4. What is the difference between type I and type II errors?
A type I error is the rejection of a true null hypothesis (i.e. a "false positive" conclusion),

WHEREAS
A type II error is the non-rejection of a false null hypothesis (i.e. a "false negative" conclusion).

Circuit 3: Improving Patient Care

You are an FY2 working on the general surgery firm. You feel that the night shift handover meeting is often rushed and unstandardised. You decide to conduct a quality improvement project for general surgery night shift handover meetings.

1. How would you plan and conduct this quality improvement project?
Good candidates will present a coherent and carefully considered plan. They should link the problem being addressed to the appropriate dimension(s) of quality in healthcare (SEPTEE: safe, effective, patient-centred, timely, efficient and equitable). They should use an appropriate framework (i.e. PDSA) in planning the QI project and state clear objectives.

2. Who would you involve in your quality improvement project?
Good candidates will present a carefully considered strategy to ensure that all key stakeholders are involved, including "who", "why", "when", "where" and "how". They will also give appropriate

examples specific to the QI project. They will not simply reel off a rehearsed list of MDT members.

3. How would you disseminate the findings of your quality improvement project?

Good candidates will present a carefully considered dissemination strategy (e.g. presenting at appropriate local/regional and national meetings, producing posters and/or digital material, and publishing a QI report using SQUIRE guidelines).

4. How could you ensure a long-term improvement in the quality of nightshift handover in general surgery after you leave the firm?

Good candidates will discuss appropriate post-intervention strategies to ensure continual, long-term improvement, e.g., registering the project with the hospital's QI/Audit department with a named consultant so that the project can be taken over by new junior doctors in future; incorporating teaching programmes as part of a regular QI session for junior doctors; working with the trust to produce working with the trust to produce guidance available online and in junior doctors' induction packs. Poor candidates will not offer any innovative ideas specific to the project.

Circuit 3: Communication Scenario

You are the Ophthalmology ST1 working in the glaucoma clinic. Your patient is a 60-year-old gentleman newly referred from the optician who suspected chronic open angle glaucoma with significant visual field loss. Your examination and visual field testing confirm this. You must communicate this diagnosis to the patient and inform him that he should inform the Driver and Vehicle Licensing Agency (DVLA) that he can no longer drive a vehicle. Please proceed to the consultation room to speak with the patient. *Briefing notes for the patient:*

- You do not think there is anything wrong with your vision. You can drive just fine.
- After hearing that you have lost your peripheral vision, you ask whether there is any treatment that can reverse the problem?
- You are worried about going blind.
- You rely on your car to get to work, do your shopping and visit your family. You do not know what you will do without being able to drive.

Good candidates will employ effective communication skills to address the ideas, concerns and expectations of the patient. Effective use of open and closed questions, active listening and empathy are required to score highly. Poor candidates will not successfully access the information in the patient's briefing notes.

Circuit 3: Clinical Knowledge Part A

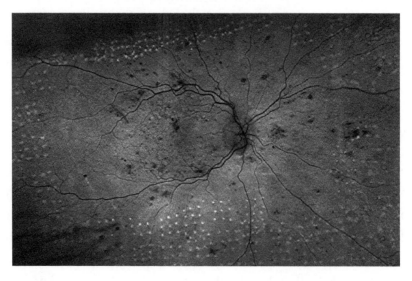

Image credit: Mr Hussein Almuhtaseb, Consultant Ophthalmic Surgeon, Bradford Royal Infirmary, UK

1. What procedure has been performed in this patient?
Panretinal photocoagulation (2 marks)

2. How does this procedure prevent the progression of diabetic retinopathy?
By destroying ischaemic retinal tissue, thereby reducing vascular endothelial growth factor (VEGF) production (2 marks)

3. List three risk factors for the progression of diabetic retinopathy.
Any three of the following (2 marks each, 6 marks max.):

- High mean HbA1c (poorly controlled diabetes mellitus)
- Long duration of diabetes mellitus
- High urine albumin-to-creatinine ratio
- Older age
- Hypertension
- Hypercholesterolaemia

4. List three classes oral drugs used in the treatment of diabetes mellitus.
Any three of the following (2 marks each, 6 marks max.):

- Alpha-glucosidase inhibitors
- Biguanides
- Dipeptidyl peptidase 4 (DPP-4) inhibitors
- Meglitinides
- Sulfonylureas
- Thiazolidinediones

Circuit 3: Clinical Knowledge Part B

A 35-year-old woman is referred to your ophthalmology clinic with the following blood test results:

Test	Result	Normal Range
TSH	<0.05 mU/l	0.5–5.5 mU/l
Thyroxine (T4)	196 nmol/l	70–140 nmol/l

5. List four systemic signs that this patient may display.
Any four of the following (2 marks each, 8 marks max.):

- Tachycardia
- Arrythmia
- Pyrexia
- Tachypnoea
- Resting tremor
- Goitre
- Thyroid acropachy (clubbing)
- Myopathy
- Pretibial myxoedema
- Skin thinning
- Increased perspiration
- Polyuria
- Amenorrhea

6. List four ocular signs that this patient may display.

Any four of the following (2 marks each, 6 marks max.):

- Lid retraction (Dalrymple's sign)
- Lid lag (Von Graefe's sign — upper lid lag on downgaze; Griffith's sign — lower lid lag on upgaze)
- Lid oedema (Enroth's sign)
- Exophthalmos
- Lagophthalmos (Stellwag's sign)
- Conjunctival injection (Goldzeiher's sign)
- Exposure keratopathy
- Increased intraocular pressure
- Restricted eye movements
- Optic neuropathy

7. Why might colour vision be affected in this patient?

Due to optic nerve compression (2 marks)

8. Name one clinical scoring system for the severity of the eye disease commonly associated with this condition.

Any one of the following (2 marks):

- Clinical Activity Score (CAS)
- Werner's Classification (NO SPECS)
- VISA Classification
- EUGOGO Classification

Circuit 3: Clinical Knowledge Part C

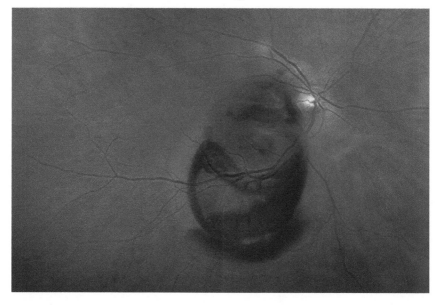

Image credit: Mr Hussein Almuhtaseb, Consultant Ophthalmic Surgeon, Bradford Royal Infirmary, UK

9. What condition is depicted in this fundus photograph?

Neovascular (wet) age-related macular degeneration (2 marks)

10. Name three risk factors for the progression of this condition.

Any three of the following (2 marks each, 6 marks max.):

- Age
- Smoking
- Female gender
- Ethnicity (Caucasian)
- Family history
- Ultraviolet (UV) light exposure
- Cardiovascular disease
- Hypertension

- Hypercholesterolaemia
- Obesity

11. Which non-invasive imaging technique helps to monitor the status of this condition?

Optical coherence tomography (2 marks)

12. Name one drug used to treat this condition.

Any one of the following (2 marks):

- Bevacizumab (Avastin)
- Ranibizumab (Lucentis)
- Aflibercept (Eylea)
- Brolucizumab (Beovu)

13. Name a landmark trial relating to the treatment of this condition.

Any one of the following (2 marks):
- Ranibizumab (Lucentis) trials:
  - ANCHOR[1]
  - MARINA[2]
  - PIER[3]
  - PrONTO[4]
- Bevacizumab (Avastin) trials:
  - CATT[5]
  - IVAN[6]

---

[1] Brown DM, *et al.* (ANCHOR study). *N Engl J Med.* 2006; 355(14):1432–44.

[2] MARINA Study Group. *N Engl J Med.* 2006; 355:1419–31.

[3] Reillo CD, *et al.* (PIER study). *Am J Ophthalmol.* 2008; 145(2):239–48.

[4] Fung AE, *et al.* (PrONTO study). *Am J Ophthalmol.* 2007; 143(4):566–83.

[5] The CATT Research Group. *N Engl J Med.* 2011; 364:1897–908.

[6] IVAN study investigators. *Lancet.* 2013; 382(9900):1258–67. doi:10.1016/ S0140-6736(13)61501-9

- Aflibercept (Eylea) trial:
  - VIEW 1 and VIEW 2[7]
  - RIVAL[8]
- Brolucizumab (Beovu) trial:
  - HAWK and HARRIER[9]

[7] VIEW 1 and VIEW 2 Study Groups. *Ophthalmology*. 2012; 119(12):2537–48. doi:10.1016/j.ophtha.2012.09.006

[8] Gillies MC, *et al.* (RIVAL study). *Ophthalmology*. 2020; 127(2):198–210. doi:10.1016/j.ophtha.2019.08.023

[9] HAWK and HARRIER Study Investigators. *Ophthalmology*. 2020; 127(1): 72–84. doi:10.1016/j.ophtha.2019.04.017

References

Note: Landmark trials for diabetic retinopathy and age-related macular degeneration are referenced as footnotes within Chapters 13 and 15, respectively.

Baile WF, Buckman R, Lenzi R, Glober G, Beale EA, Kudelka, AP. SPIKES — A six-step protocol for delivering bad news: application to the patient with cancer. *Oncologist*. 2000; 5:302–11. doi:10.1634/theoncologist.5-4-302

Batalden PB, Davidoff F. What is "quality improvement" and how can it transform healthcare? *BMJ Quality & Safety*. 2007; 16:2–3.

CASP. CASP checklists. 2020. https://casp-uk.net/casp-tools-checklists/. Accessed 2 June 2020.

Cochrane. *Cochrane Handbook for Systematic Reviews of Interventions*. Version 6.1, 2020. https://training.cochrane.org/handbook. Accessed November 2020.

Fisher LD, Dixon DO, Herson J, Frankowski RK, Hearron MS, Peace KE. Intention to treat in clinical trials. In: *Statistical Issues In Drug Research and Development*. Peace KE, editor. New York: Marcel Dekker; 1990. pp. 331–50.

Gillam S, Siriwardena AN. Frameworks for improvement: clinical audit, the plan-do-study-act cycle and significant event audit. *Qual Prim Care*. 2013; 21(2):123–30.

Health Education England. Expenses policy for candidates attending interviews for medical or dental training programmes. 2020. https://specialtytraining. hee.nhs.uk/portals/1/Content/Resource%20Bank/Expenses/Candidate%20 Expenses%20Policy.pdf. Accessed 25 June 2020.

Institute of Medicine. *Crossing the Quality Chasm: A New Health System for the 21st Century*. Washington DC: National Academy Press, 1990, p. 244.

Kurtz S, Silverman J, Benson J, Draper J. Marrying content and process in clinical method teaching: enhancing the Calgary–Cambridge guides. *Acad Med*. 2003; 78(8):802–9. doi:10.1097/00001888-200308000-00011

Marsden, AJ. Empathetic consultation skills in undergraduate medical education: a qualitative approach. 2014. PhD Thesis. University of East Anglia, Norwich Medical School. https://ueaeprints.uea.ac.uk/id/eprint/49603/1/2014Marsden.pdf. Accessed December 2020.

NHS Improvement. Stakeholder analysis. 2018. https://improvement.nhs.uk/documents/2169/stakeholder-analysis.pdf. Accessed June 2020.

NICE. Principles for best practice in clinical audit. 2002. https://www.nice.org.uk/media/default/About/what-we-do/Into-practice/principles-for-best-practice-in-clinical-audit.pdf. Accessed 3 June 2020.

Royal College of Ophthalmologists. 2020a. National recruitment for ophthalmic specialist training. https://www.rcophth.ac.uk/training/national-recruitment-ophthalmic-specialist-training/. Accessed November 2020.

Royal College of Ophthalmologists. 2020b. Eyesi ophthalmic surgical simulators in the UK & Ireland. https://www.rcophth.ac.uk/training/ost-information/simulation/eyesi-ophthalmic-surgical-simulators-in-the-uk-ireland/. Accessed November 2020.

Severn Postgraduate Medical Education. 2020a. Ophthalmology. https://severndeanery.nhs.uk/recruitment/vacancies/show/oph-st1-2021. Accessed November 2020.

Severn Postgraduate Medical Education. 2020b. Interview guidance. 2020. https://severndeanery.nhs.uk/recruitment/vacancies/show/ophth-1-2020/interview-guidance-lib. Accessed 25 June 2020.

SQUIRE. Revised standards for quality improvement reporting excellence: SQUIRE 2.0. 2017. http://squire-statement.org/index.cfm?fuseaction=Page.ViewPage&PageID=471. Accessed July 2020.

World Health Organization. *WHO Recommendations on the Diagnosis of HIV Infection in Infants and Children*. Geneva: World Health Organization; 2010. ANNEX 4, Characteristics of a screening test. https://www.ncbi.nlm.nih.gov/books/NBK138555/. Accessed July 2020.

Yemm G (2013). *Essential Guide to Leading Your Team: How to Set Goals, Measure Performance and Reward Talent*. Pearson Education, pp. 37–9.

Acknowledgements

I would like to thank the following:

Prof. I Christopher Lloyd for kindly reviewing this book, writing the foreword, providing the external cataract photograph and support and encouragement.

Mr Hussein Almuhtaseb for kindly providing fundus photographs using the Optomap retinal imaging device (Optos plc, Dunfermline, UK) and support and encouragement.

All my colleagues, supervisors, mentors and patients for introducing me to the art and science of ophthalmology — it is a privilege to continue learning from you all.

World Scientific Publishing for publishing this book.

Index